Professor Khan would like to dedicate this work to Heinke, Jani
and Zarie.

Contents

Steps of a systematic review

Case studies

● *Preface*

Are you a health professional who wishes to improve the quality of your practice using systematic reviews? Are you embarking on a career in public health, epidemiology or health technology assessment? Are you a clinical teacher interested in discovering the likely educational effects of the courses you deliver? Are you interested in health from the social science perspective? Are you about to start your first review? If so, this book is for you.

The first edition of this book exceeded all expectations. It was commended in the Basis of Medicine category in the BMA Medical Book competition 2003. Commentators found it a clear, useful guide to a potentially off-putting topic that built the confidence of non-statisticians. The *British Journal of Surgery* called it a 'gem'. It recognized that it stood head and shoulders above other texts on account of its brevity and clarity of prose. It advised readers that if they ever read or wrote systematic reviews, they should read this book first. It was praised for conveying an enthusiasm that made the reader want to conduct a review of their own. Its well-organized materials, logical structured flow and useful worked examples led to a recommendation to all libraries of educational and research institutions concerned with health sciences. It was directed at novice reviewers, but it was cited over a hundred times, indicating that even seasoned researchers took quite an interest in its contents. With the passage of time a second edition became imperative. Like the first, this edition describes the main principles behind systematic reviews of healthcare research and provides guidance on how reviews can be appraised, conducted and applied in practice.

As our current healthcare practice and policy increasingly relies on clear and comprehensive summaries of information collated through systematic literature reviews, it is necessary for us to understand how reviews and practice guidelines are produced. You may not be trained in health research methods, but this book will enable you to grasp the principles behind reviewing literature. In this way you will be able to critically appraise published systematic reviews and guidelines, and evaluate their inferences and recommendations for application in your practice.

Published reviews and guidelines are not always adequate or sufficient for our needs. Have you ever wondered how you could conduct your own review? The resources required for undertaking reviews are increasingly becoming available in a clinical setting. The appointment of clinical librarians, internet access to many journals, ease of obtaining interlibrary loans and the availability of user-friendly software make it possible for systematic reviews to be conducted by healthcare practitioners. This book highlights the core information necessary for planning and preparing reviews. It focuses on a clinical readership and new reviewers, not on experienced epidemiologists, social scientists, medical educationalists and statisticians. Using this book you will be able to initiate your own review.

What is new in this edition of the book? We have widened the scope to go beyond evaluation of effectiveness of interventions in healthcare. We demonstrate how reviews can be usefully applied to evaluate qualitative and educational research. We have thoroughly overhauled the section and examples on how to interpret the findings of a review, leading to judicious and credible recommendations for clinical practice. We have added a substantial number of new case studies, providing more worked illustration of key concepts.

For too many years there has been a mystery surrounding systematic reviews and reviewers. How did they select certain studies and reject others? What did they do to collate results? How did a bunch of insignificant findings suddenly become significant? You are about to embark on a journey that will demystify these intrigues. Enjoy reading.

KS Khan,
R Kunz,
J Kleijnen,
G Antes

● *About the authors*

Together we are veterans of over 250 systematic reviews. Over the years we have worked with healthcare commissioners, clinicians and other decision makers, producing reviews to inform policy and practice. We have collaborated with other epidemiologists and statisticians to advance methods for undertaking systematic reviews. Two of us work in an academic setting producing and promoting systematic reviews; two of us work in a clinical setting with patients, applying evidence from reviews to inform our practice.

Khalid S Khan is the Professor of Women's Health and Clinical Epidemiology at Bart and the London Medical School in Queen Mary, University of London. He is a clinician, trained in systematic reviews and evidence-based medicine (EBM). Qualified in medical education, he runs journal club and other EBM activities, including evidence-supported ward rounds and workshops on critical appraisal. As a clinical academic he leads a number of systematic review projects, teaches undergraduates and postgraduates, and provides peer review to several clinical journals.

Regina Kunz has recently been appointed Director of the Institute for Insurance Medicine at the University and University Hospital Basel, Switzerland. Nephrologist and clinical epidemiologist by training, she has comprehensive expertise in doing systematic reviews, meta-analyses and health technology assessments. Then, her clinical practice reminded her day by day how important it is to have high quality evidence syntheses at hand when advising patients and making management decisions. Today, the lack of high quality evidence synthesis in insurance medicine is a painful experience that urgently needs change. Her academic activities within the Grading of Recommendations Assessment, Development and Evaluation (GRADE) working group on guideline methodology and as a long-standing board member of the Guidelines International Network G-I-N corroborate the need for high quality reviews and meta-analyses in all areas of healthcare, to provide physicians, patients and decision makers with sound recommendations, and the difficulties of delivering convincing recommendations in the absence of such reviews. She is the founding member of the German Network EbM, editor of the German textbook Evidence-based Medicine in Clinic and Practice, and has a great deal of experience in running teaching courses on systematic reviews and meta-analyses, the GRADE-methodology and evidence-based medicine worldwide.

Jos Kleijnen is the Director of an independent company, Kleijnen Systematic Reviews Ltd and Professor of Systematic Reviews in Health Care at Maastricht University. Following his graduation from medical school, he pursued a career as a clinical epidemiologist and has a wealth of experience in conducting and disseminating systematic reviews and other research. He is a member of various steering groups and advisory committees related to systematic reviews and health technology assessment. He was the founding Director of the Dutch Cochrane Centre, Professor and Director of the Centre for Reviews and Dissemination at the University of York, and is a member of several Methods Working Groups of the Cochrane Collaboration. He is an editor of the Cochrane Peripheral Vascular Diseases Review Group and also teaches on courses on systematic reviews and EBM in several countries. This includes a collaboration with the Horten Centre in Zurich and with the Vienna School of Clinical Research in Vienna.

Gerd Antes is the Director of the German Cochrane Centre, Freiburg. He is a medical statistician and has in-depth knowledge of the mathematics behind meta-analyses, heterogeneity, funnel plots, etc. As well as his interests in methodological work, statistical computing and medical informatics, he set up the German Cochrane initiative and spends considerable time supporting the progress of EBM and systematic reviews. He has been a founding member and previous president of the German EBM Network. He has also been a member of the Cochrane Collaboration Steering Group for several years. He is a member of the German Committee for Clinical Guidelines and of the German Commission for Vaccination. One of his activities includes teaching and training science journalists. He has also successfully contributed to the establishment of the German Register for Clinical Trials.

We have put this book together because we feel that health professionals have much to gain from reviews and guidelines and, at the same time, reviews and guidelines have much to gain from them. With this book we hope healthcare practitioners will feel empowered to use reviews effectively and to initiate their own reviews.

Acknowledgements

No work can ever be completed without the support of many. The authors are grateful to Susan Hahné, Anjum Doshani, Peter J Thompson and Jack Cohen for their critical review of an earlier version of this book; Mary Publicover for her review of Step 2; Christine Anne Clark and Anne-Marie Bagnall for their review of Case study 1; Sue O'Meara for her review of Case study 3; Elaine Denny for her contribution to Case study 5; Sharon Buckley for her contribution to Case study 6; and Katja Suter for her contribution to Case studies 7 and 8.

● *Abbreviations*

BEME	Best Evidence Medical Education Collaboration
CCTR	Cochrane Controlled Trials Register (this is now called CENTRAL)
CDSR	Cochrane Database of Systematic Reviews
CER	Control Event Rate
CI	Confidence Interval
DARE	Database of Abstracts of Reviews of Effects
EBM	Evidence-based Medicine
EER	Experimental Event Rate
ES	Effect Size (for continuous data)
GRADE	The Grading of Recommendations Assessment, Development and Evaluation working group
HTA	Health Technology Assessment
ITT	Intention-to-treat Analysis
LR	Likelihood Ratio (LR+, LR for positive test result; LR–, LR for negative test result)
MeSH	Medical Subject Heading
NNT	Number Needed to Treat
OR	Odds Ratio (*not to be confused with Boolean operator OR used in searching literature electronically*)
RCT	Randomized Controlled Trial
RD	Risk Difference (or ARR, absolute risk reduction)
RR	Relative Risk
SD	Standard Deviation
SE	Standard Error

Introduction

We hardly ever come across a healthcare journal that does not publish reviews. All disciplines related to medicine, including social science and medical education, rely heavily on reviews for guiding practice and scholarship. What makes them ubiquitous? Reviews provide summaries of evidence contained in a number of individual studies on a specific topic. Research that is relevant to our practice is scattered all over the literature and sometimes it is published in languages foreign to us. By going through a single review article in our own language we can get a quick overview of a wide range of evidence on a particular topic. Therefore, we like reviews. They provide us with a way of keeping up-to-date without the trouble of having to go through the individual studies relevant to our practice. With an ever-increasing number of things to do in our professional lives and not enough time to do them, who wouldn't find reviews handy? In all honesty, even if we had the time and means to identify and appraise relevant studies, many of us would still prefer reviews.

Now a word of warning – the manner in which traditional reviews search for studies, collate evidence and generate inferences is often suspect. In the worst cases, personal interests of the author may drive the whole of the review process and its conclusions. After all, many of the reviews we read are invited commentaries; they are not properly conducted pieces of research. So, how can we be certain that reviews are not misleading us? This is why systematic reviews have come to replace traditional reviews.

Robust systematic reviews of healthcare literature are proper pieces of research. They identify relevant studies, appraise their quality and summarize their results using scientific methodology. In this way they differ from traditional reviews and off-the-cuff commentaries produced by 'experts'. More importantly, the recommendations of systematic reviews, instead of reflecting personal views of 'experts', are based on balanced inferences generated from the collated evidence.

This book describes the principles behind systematically reviewing the literature on healthcare and related subjects. Using this book, readers should be able to confidently appraise a review for its quality, as well as initiate one of their own.

Critically appraising systematic reviews

More and more healthcare policy is being based on clear and comprehensive summaries of information collated through systematic reviews of the relevant literature. So, in the current day and age, evidence-based practice requires more than just critical

A **systematic review** is a research article that identifies relevant studies, appraises their quality and summarizes their results using a scientific methodology.

The term **meta-analysis** is not synonymous with a **systematic review**. It is only a part of the **review**. It is a statistical technique for combining the results of a number of individual studies to produce a summary result. Some publications called meta-analysis are not systematic reviews.

From here onwards, whenever this book uses the term **review**, it will mean a **systematic review**, using these terms interchangeably. Reviews should never be done in any other way.

Meta-synthesis is the synthesis of existing qualitative research findings on a specific research question. This does not involve meta-analysis.

Evidence-based medicine (EBM) is the judicious use of current best evidence in making decisions about healthcare. Systematic reviews provide strong evidence to underpin EBM.

appraisal of individual studies. Practice guidelines are a prime example of how systematic reviews have come to occupy a pivotal role in our professional lives.

Systematic reviews may represent a quantum leap in review methodology. However, we should not have blind faith. Reviews and guidelines, just like individual studies, can be of a variable quality. There are numerous examples of poor reviews published in top healthcare journals and of inferior guidelines produced by professional bodies. Hence, there is a potential for misleading inferences even among apparently robust reviews and guidelines. Therefore, it is necessary for us, as healthcare practitioners, to acquire a deeper understanding of the principles behind systematic reviews. Although we may only have a basic knowledge in health research methods and consider the task of appraising reviews onerous, with this book, readers will be able to grasp the process and pitfalls of systematically reviewing literature, and discriminate between robust and not-so-robust reviews and guidelines more easily.

We can identify existing reviews to support our practice by searching the resources shown in Box 0.1. Once relevant reviews have been identified, the quality of their methods should be appraised, their evidence should be examined and their findings should be assessed for application in practice. Examples of how to use findings from existing reviews are shown in the case studies in Section B of this book. When drawing on reviews to support our practice, we will occasionally become painfully aware that relevant reviews either do not exist or they supply inadequate information. When you can't find a review that meets your needs, why not initiate a new one?

Guidelines are systematically developed statements to assist practitioners and patients in making decisions about specific clinical situations. They often, but not always, use evidence from systematic reviews.

What is involved in the identification, appraisal and application of evidence summarized in reviews?

Framing questions
|
Identifying relevant reviews
|
Assessing quality of the review and its evidence
|
Summarizing the evidence
|
Interpreting the findings

Box 0.1 Selected sources of systematic reviews and guidelines

The Cochrane Library* (www.thecochranelibrary.com) has several databases of published and ongoing systematic reviews:

- **The Cochrane Database of Systematic Reviews (CDSR)**
  Contains the full text of regularly updated systematic reviews of healthcare interventions carried out by the Cochrane Collaboration, plus protocols for reviews currently in preparation.
- **Database of Abstracts of Reviews of Effects (DARE)⁺**
  Critical appraisals of systematic reviews found in sources other than CDSR. These reviews are identified by regular searching of bibliographic databases, hand searching of key major medical journals, and scanning grey literature.
- **Health Technology Assessment (HTA) Database⁺**
  Abstracts of completed technology assessments and ongoing projects being conducted by members of the International Network of Agencies for Health Technology Assessment (INAHTA) and other healthcare technology agencies. Most of these include systematic reviews.

- **Collaborative Review Groups (CRGs)**
  Found under 'about the Cochrane Collaboration' in the Cochrane Library. It contains a list of the total output of each one of 95 CRGs and provides an alternative method of searching the Cochrane Library.

There are more systematic reviews around than one might think. For example, in the 2nd issue of the 2011 Cochrane Library alone there were 6671 complete reviews and protocols combined in April 2011, 14602 abstracts of quality assessed reviews in DARE and 9965 abstracts of technology assessments in the HTA database.

General electronic databases: (*also see Box 2.3*)

- MEDLINE – PubMed Clinical Queries using the Systematic Reviews feature available at www.ncbi.nlm.nih.gov/entrez/query/static/clinical.html. At the time of writing there were 126 190 citations included in the PubMed Systematic Reviews subset strategy.
- CINAHL, EMBASE, PsycLIT and others may be searched for reviews by adapting one of the search filters (a combination of text words, indexing terms and subject headings that captures relevant articles) available from the Centre for Reviews and Dissemination search strategies available at http://www.york.ac.uk/inst/crd/identifying_research_evidence.htm

Selected internet sites:

- CMA Infobase – Clinical Practice Guidelines – www.mdm.ca/cpgsnew/cpgs/index.asp
- Guidelines and Guidelines in Practice – www.eguidelines.co.uk
- GIN Guidelines International Network – www.g-i-n.org:
- HTA Programme of the National Institute for Health Research (NIHR) – www.ncchta.org/project/htapubs.asp
- NHS Evidence – http://www.evidence.nhs.uk/nhs-evidence-content/journals-and-databases
- National Institute for Health and Clinical Excellence (NICE) – www.nice.org.uk/
- OMNI – www.omni.ac.uk (use advanced search and specify Practice Guidelines in Resource Type)
- International Prospective Register of Systematic Reviews (PROSPERO) http://www.crd.york.ac.uk/PROSPERO/
- ScHARR-Lock's Guide to the evidence – www.shef.ac.uk/uni/academic/R-Z/scharr/ir/scebm.html
- SIGN guidelines – http://www.sign.ac.uk/index.html
- Turning Research Into Practice (TRIP) – www.tripdatabase.com

Selected print publications:

- Clinical Evidence – www.clinicalevidence.org

*See Case study 1 for an example search of the Cochrane Library
⁺Also available free at http://www.york.ac.uk/inst/crd

Web sites are constantly changing. The internet addresses provided in this book were obtained from searches in June 2011.

Conducting a systematic review

Internet access to literature searching, the ability to obtain articles either electronically or through interlibrary loans, user-friendly software for meta-analysis, etc. all make this kind of reviewing possible. As these resources are increasingly available in a clinical setting, undertaking systematic reviews has become a realistic option for healthcare practitioners. But why should practitioners undertake reviews?

There is no shortage of reasons for undertaking one's own review. One may wish to conduct reviews for supporting evidence-based practice, personal professional development, informing clinical policy, publishing in a peer-reviewed journal, writing an introduction to a research thesis, or preparing a presentation at a conference, a technical report or an invited commentary.

However, there should be no need to reinvent the wheel. Existing reviews and guidelines should be used to their full potential. Up-to-date good quality reviews may already contain all the information we need.

When reviews and guidelines on a specific topic do not exist, are not up-to-date or are of a poor quality, our options are:

- ask 'experts' for advice
- appraise available primary studies
- conduct a systematic review.

We realize that 'expert' opinions may not be evidence-based and they may be unacceptable to others – for every 'expert' there is an equal and opposite 'expert'. We know that appraisal of individual studies will not provide information on the complete picture. Isn't this the point where we want to start a new review? Many Cochrane reviews commence in this way and when they are published everyone can benefit from them. Conducting a new systematic review will take a lot of effort, but not everything that is worthwhile is easy.

When undertaking research projects, advanced courses or educational assignments, we (or at least our supervisors) should be aware that non-systematic reviews are increasingly less acceptable. Where do we go next? We should do our own systematic review. As academics in the health professions (without advanced epidemiology and statistics training), we may be used to publishing editorials, opinions and commentaries. We are now under pressure from journal editors to be more systematic in our approach. Why not try a systematic review for the next commentary? We may feel inhibited as the knowledge or skills required for initiating such reviews may not be within our grasp. Help is in our hands. This book provides the core information necessary for planning and initiating reviews of healthcare literature.

This book focuses primarily on a clinical readership and first-time reviewers, not on epidemiologists, social scientists, educationalists and statisticians. This book will enable readers

The **Cochrane Collaboration**, established in 1993, is an international network of people helping healthcare providers, policy makers, patients, their advocates and carers, make well-informed decisions about human health care by preparing, updating and promoting the accessibility of **Cochrane** Reviews

Cochrane Reviews are systematic reviews of primary research in human health care and health policy. They investigate the effects of interventions (literally meaning to intervene to modify an outcome) for prevention, treatment and rehabilitation. They also assess the accuracy of a diagnostic test for a given condition in a specific patient group and setting.

to initiate reviews without relying on professional reviewers and will also give advice about further reading and how to seek professional input in difficult areas. Considering the nature of work involved in the various Steps of a review, it is advisable to find one or more other reviewers to join in. First-time reviewers might want to attend a local workshop or course on systematic reviews. The Cochrane Collaboration organizes many of these – why not ask the local Cochrane Centre about their next training event?

How this book is structured

This book will help readers to understand the principles of systematic reviews. In the discourse that follows there is a step-by-step explanation of the review process. There are just five steps. This book provides guidance for each step of a review with examples from published reviews. Many examples are followed through the different steps so that we will be able to see the link between the steps. In addition, application of the theory is illustrated through case studies. Each case consists of a scenario requiring evidence from reviews, a demonstration of some review methods and a proposed resolution of the scenario. Insight into critical appraisal and conducting a systematic review can be gained by working through the various Steps, examples and case studies.

If we have made up our mind to initiate a review, we should first produce a brief outline (or a protocol) of the project, giving some background information and a specification of the problem to be addressed along with the methodology to be used in the review. Throughout the review work, the protocol will remind us where we are coming from and what direction we want to go in, avoiding distractions and keeping us on track. It will also provide a document that could be peer reviewed before the review work is commenced. Some people suggest that a review protocol should be posted on a website to facilitate a wide peer review, but input from visitors to the site may be variable. Realistically, we have a much better chance of getting a professional to comment on the protocol if we ask a colleague experienced in reviewing or if we register our review with a relevant Review Group of the Cochrane or the Best Evidence Medical Education (BEME) Collaboration.

This book will be a useful companion in protocol development as well as throughout the five steps in the review process:

- First, the problems to be addressed have to be specified in the form of well-structured questions (Step 1). This is a key step, as all other aspects of the review follow directly from the questions.
- Second, thorough literature searches have to be conducted to identify potentially relevant studies which can shed light on the questions (Step 2). This is an essential feature that makes a review systematic.
- Third, the quality of the selected studies is assessed (Step 3).

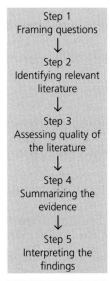

Step 1
Framing questions
↓
Step 2
Identifying relevant literature
↓
Step 3
Assessing quality of the literature
↓
Step 4
Summarizing the evidence
↓
Step 5
Interpreting the findings

The **Best Evidence in Medical Education (BEME)** Collaboration is committed to the promotion of BEME through the dissemination and production of systematic reviews of medical education. An additional objective is the creation of a culture of BEME amongst teachers, institutions and national bodies.

- Fourth, the evidence concerning study characteristics and results is summarized (Step 4). When feasible and appropriate, statistical meta-analysis helps in collating results.
- Finally, inferences and recommendations for practice are generated by interpreting and exploring the clinical relevance of the findings (Step 5).

The key points about appraisal and conduct of reviews are summarized at the end of each Step in Section A of this book. The case studies in Section B illustrate the application of the review theory that is covered in the five Steps. Readers may prefer to assimilate the review theory before turning to the case studies or they may read them in conjunction with the information contained in the first section. A 'suggested reading' list provides references to direct readers to other texts for theoretical and methodological issues that are beyond the core material covered in this book.

> This book will focus mainly on reviews of research, examining the effects of *interventions* or *exposures* on *outcomes*.

The guidance in this book is pitched at a level suitable for users of systematic reviews and for novice reviewers. It should not be seen as providing a 'set menu' for appraising and undertaking systematic reviews. What it offers is a range of 'à la carte' guidance, which can be applied flexibly depending on the question and context.

Key points about this book

- This book will enable readers to confidently appraise published reviews for their quality, as well as to initiate their own reviews.
- It describes the main principles behind systematically reviewing literature on the effects of healthcare, focusing on a readership of healthcare professionals.
- It includes a step-by-step explanation of how to appraise and conduct reviews along with illustrative examples and case studies.
- Key points about critical appraisal and conduct of a review are summarized at the end of each Step.

Section A: *Steps of a systematic review*

This section provides a step-by-step explanation of the processes involved when carrying out a review. There are just five Steps. For each Step, basic principles of a review are explained, using examples from published reviews. Many examples are followed through the different steps so that readers will be able to see the link between the various stages.

Step 1: Framing questions for a review

▼

Step 2: Identifying relevant literature

▼

Step 3: Assessing the quality of the literature

▼

Step 4: Summarizing the evidence

▼

Step 5: Interpreting the findings

● Step 1: *Framing questions for a review*

Systematic reviews are carried out to generate answers to focused questions about healthcare and related issues. The key to a successful review project lies in the reviewer's ability to be precise and specific when stating the problems to be addressed in the review. This is a critical part of the review because, as will become apparent in subsequent Steps, all other aspects of the review flow directly from the original questions. In this Step, we will consider the question formulation process in detail and briefly look at the thinking required to examine the potential impact of variations in the different components of a review question.

1.1 An approach to formulating questions

Formulating questions is not as easy as it may sound. A structured approach to framing questions, which uses four components or facets, may be used. These components include the *populations*, *interventions* (or *exposures*), and *outcomes* related to the problem posed in the review, and the *designs* of studies that are suitable for addressing it. We can see the relationship between the various question components in the comparative study in Box 1.1.

After reading Box 1.1, the formulation of questions will probably seem like a daunting task to new reviewers. We may begin to have second thoughts, but we should not give up – help is at hand. This chapter of the book will take us through the question formulation process so that our review can have just the right start. It is well-recognized that even quite experienced clinicians don't always find it easy to frame questions for evidence-based practice, so new reviewers can also expect to have a rough ride during the initial stages of their reviews. It will take some effort, but its value will be realized soon, as the rest of the review will flow directly and efficiently from the questions.

Most serious reviewers devote a substantial amount of time and effort in getting the questions right before embarking on a review. They do this because they want to avoid having to change questions later on during the review. We should make no exceptions. If there is any difficulty in figuring out the components of questions, we should first write them down in free form. We can then reconstruct the free form question into a structured format as exemplified in Box 1.2.

We should think of a *population* as a description of the group of participants or patients about whom evidence is being sought in the review. Imagine *interventions* as the actions or the alternatives being considered for the *population*. *Outcomes* are measures of

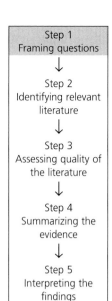

Step 1
Framing questions
↓
Step 2
Identifying relevant literature
↓
Step 3
Assessing quality of the literature
↓
Step 4
Summarizing the evidence
↓
Step 5
Interpreting the findings

Question components
- The populations
- The interventions
- The outcomes
- The study designs

Free form question: It describes the query for which one seeks an answer through a review in simple language (however vague).

Structured question: Reviewers convert free form questions into a clear and explicit format using a structured approach (see Box 1.2). This makes the query potentially answerable through existing relevant studies.

Box 1.1 Framing structured questions for systematic reviews

Question components

- The populations

  Succinct description of a group of participants or patients, their clinical problem and the healthcare setting.

- The interventions (or exposures)

  The main action(s) being considered, e.g. treatments, processes of care, social intervention, educational intervention, risk factors, tests, etc.

- The outcomes

  The clinical changes in health state (morbidity, mortality) and other related changes, e.g. health resource use.

- The study design

  The appropriate ways to recruit participants or patients in a research study, give them interventions and measure their outcomes.

Relationship between the question components in a comparative study

A comparative study assesses the effect of an intervention using comparison groups. For example, it may allocate participants or patients (with or without randomization) from a relevant *population* to alternative groups of *interventions* (or *exposures*) and follow them up to determine the effect of the *interventions* (or *exposures*) on *outcome*.

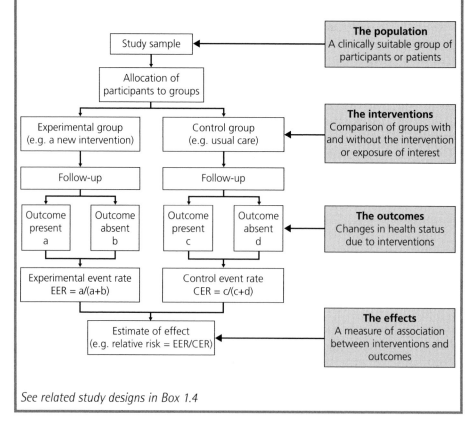

See related study designs in Box 1.4

Box 1.2 Some example questions

An example question about clinical effectiveness

Free form question: Which of the many available antimicrobial products improve healing in patients with chronic wounds?

Structured question

● The population	In adults with various forms of chronic wounds in an ambulatory setting ....
● The interventions	.... would systemic or topical antimicrobial preparations ....
● The outcomes	.... improve wound healing?
● The study design	A comparative study that allocates subjects with chronic wounds to alternative therapeutic interventions of interest and determines the effect of the interventions on wound healing (e.g. randomized controlled trial).

See Case study 3 for a related review

An example question about aetiology

Free form question: Is exposure to benzodiazepines in pregnancy associated with malformations in the newborn baby?

Structured question

● The population	In pregnant women ....
● The exposures	.... does exposure to benzodiazepines during early pregnancy ....
● The outcomes	.... cause malformations in the newborn baby?
● The study designs	● A study that recruits women in early pregnancy, assesses their exposure to benzodiazepines, follows them up and examines their newborn babies to compare the rates of malformations among women with exposure and those without (cohort study).
	● A study that retrospectively compares exposure to benzodiazepines in early pregnancy among women who have given birth to a child with malformation with those women who gave birth to a healthy child (case-control study).

See Box 5.2 for a related meta-analysis

An example question about test accuracy

Free form question: Among postmenopausal women with abnormal vaginal bleeding, does pelvic ultrasound scan exclude uterine cancer accurately?

Structured question

● The population	In postmenopausal women, within a community setting, with vaginal bleeding ....
● The test	.... does a uterine ultrasound scan test accurately predict ....
● The reference standard	.... histological diagnosis of uterine cancer?

● The study design	A study that recruits women from a relevant population, uses the test (scan) and a reference standard investigation to confirm or refute the presence of cancer (histology), and determines the accuracy with which the test identifies cancer (*see Box C4.3*).

See Case study 4 for a related review

An example question about qualitative research

Free form question: How does the experience of endometriosis impact on women's lives?

Structured question

● The population	In women with a confirmed diagnosis of endometriosis....
● The intervention	.... how does observation or treatment....
● The outcomes	.... affect pain, social relationships and self-image?
● The study design	A study that narrates subjective experiences (*see Box C5.3*).

See Case study 5 for a related review

An example question about an educational intervention

Free form question: How does use of portfolios affect student learning in undergraduate (medical and nursing) education?

Structured question

● The population	Among undergraduate nursing or medical students ....
● The intervention	.... does a 'portfolio', defined as a collection of evidence of student learning, a learning journal or diary, or a combination of these two elements ....
● The outcomes	.... improve knowledge and skills?
● The study design	A study that evaluates the educational effects of portfolios.

See Case study 6 for a related review

what the *population* wants to achieve from the *interventions*, e.g. avoiding illness or death. Finally, we should think of how a worthwhile study could be *designed* to examine the effect of the *interventions*. For example, by comparing *outcomes* between groups of a *population* with and without the *intervention*, the effect may be assessed in terms of illness avoided by use of an *intervention*.

The point about question formulation is that a structured approach should be used. The structure outlined in Box 1.1 should never become a 'straight jacket' and it may be modified to meet the needs of our free form question, depending on where our interest in healthcare lies. For example, in epidemiology the questions may be about aetiology. We can easily substitute the component *interventions* with *exposure* and frame the questions in terms of how *outcomes* might be different in *populations* exposed or not exposed to certain agents or risk factors (Box 1.2). For questions

Section A of this book will focus mainly on questions relating to **quantitative** effects of *interventions* (therapy, prevention, social care, etc.) or *exposures* (environmental agents, risk factors, etc.) in the context of **comparative** *study designs*.

Section B of this book will also cover systematic reviews of qualitative and educational research.

about the accuracy of screening or diagnostic tests we might substitute the component *intervention* with *test*, and *outcome* with *reference standard* against which the accuracy of the *test* will be measured (Box 1.2). In this way the proposed structure is versatile and adaptable for a wide range of question types.

1.2 Variations in populations, interventions and outcomes

Once the way in which questions are structured is understood (Box 1.1), we should be able to see that systematic reviews are analyses of existing studies within a given set of *populations*, *interventions* and *outcomes*. We may have started with some scepticism about framing our question in this way; however, with the realization that different *populations*, *interventions* and *outcomes* exist within our free form question, we are likely to end up with many more than one question. If we have not, we should look hard to see if there is some variation within each of our question components. This is critical – even in a straightforward question about antimicrobials for chronic wounds (Box 1.2), it should be clear that there are many types of chronic wounds (*populations*), antimicrobials (*interventions*) and ways of measuring wound healing (*outcomes*) (Box 1.3).

It is important to seriously consider how *populations*, *interventions* and *outcomes* might vary among existing studies. Such differences are important in defining study selection criteria (Step 2) and planning the tabulation of findings (Steps 4 and 5). They are also relevant in understanding the reasons for variation in effects of *interventions* from study to study (Step 4) and in exploring the strength of the evidence to gauge applicability of the findings (Step 5). Thus, conclusions of individual studies and reviews may vary depending on differences in the characteristics of their *populations*, the nature or delivery of their *interventions* and the types of *outcomes*. These issues are examined in detail later on in the book. Here we briefly examine their implications when framing questions.

1.2.1 Variations in populations

Population characteristics may vary between studies with respect to patients' age and sex, severity of illness, presence of co-existing illnesses, etc. For instance, when the effect of home visits is studied among elderly people (Box 1.3), the *intervention* is effective among young–old rather than old–old people (Box 4.5).

1.2.2 Variations in interventions

The *intervention* features such as the care setting, compliance or intensity, additional routine care, etc. may also be associated with variable effects. For example, among elderly people, home visits are more effective if multidimensional assessments are used and follow-up is frequent (Box 4.5). Defining the comparator is a critical element. If we wish to compare drug A *versus* drug B, we should be clear about this. The literature may only provide studies comparing drug A *versus* placebo and drug B *versus* placebo. This will amount to an indirect comparison, a deviation from our focus on the effectiveness of drug A assessed directly against drug B.

1.2.3 Variations in outcomes

We need to identify all clinically relevant *outcomes*, which will help in examining the success or failure of the *interventions*. During our review it may become apparent that existing studies have not directly measured *outcomes* we felt were critical and important. Identification of these deficiencies in existing studies is important by itself for transparency in reviews.

A relevant *outcome* is one that directly measures issues of importance to the population. Often these data cannot be easily acquired, and there may be a tendency, both among reviewers and readers, to become interested in intermediate, surrogate or proxy *outcome* measurements. For example, when we are really interested in discovering the effect of fluoride therapy in preventing fractures, we might be tempted to investigate bone mineral content as a surrogate *outcome*, as it would be easier to obtain information about this. How misleading such an approach can be is demonstrated in a randomized controlled trial (*N Engl J Med* 1999; **322**: 802–9); bone density increased significantly (10–35% at different skeletal sites as compared to placebo) among the participants treated with fluorides; however, there was a nearly three-fold increase in non-vertebral fractures (control 24 *vs* fluorides 72, *p* = 0.01), which was unexpected. This makes it evident that conclusions from research based on surrogate *outcomes* are likely to be weak when it comes to making decisions in practice. As we delineate in Step 5, the strength and weakness of evidence should be evaluated separately for each outcome, even when data come from the same studies. Therefore it is crucial that *outcomes* are set out in detail at the outset in a review.

When considering the *outcomes* for a review question, we should think about what we mean by health. Is it just the absence of illness or disease? This section of the book mainly focuses on quantitative morbidity or mortality *outcomes*. In the next section we also demonstrate how reviews collate evidence on *outcomes* used in qualitative and educational research (Case studies 5 and 6). It has become fashionable to consider the question of how to achieve optimal *outcomes* with the smallest input of resources. This allows us to discover whether the investment in *interventions* is likely to be worthwhile. In this situation *outcomes* need to focus on the costs of providing healthcare in addition to clinical *outcomes* (Box 1.3). We will not cover these value-for-money issues much beyond framing the questions.

Clinically relevant *outcomes* directly measure what is important to patients in terms of how they feel, what their function is, and whether they survive.

Surrogate *outcome* measurements substitute for direct outcome measures. They include physiological variables or measures of subclinical disease. To be valid, the surrogate must be statistically correlated with the clinically relevant outcome.

Box 1.3 Framing questions for reviews: Variations in *population, interventions, outcomes* and *study designs*

Three example questions about clinical effectiveness

Free form question: Which of the many available antimicrobial products improve healing in patients with chronic wounds?

Structured question *(expanded from Box 1.2)*

● The population	Adults with various forms of chronic wounds:	● Diabetic ulcers ● Venous ulcers ● Pressure ulcers
● The interventions	Antimicrobial preparations: *versus* Comparator:	● Systemic preparations ● Topical preparations *versus* ● Other preparations
● The outcomes	Various measures to quantify improvement in a critical outcome 'wound healing':	● Outcome measured directly: Complete healing, amputation due to wound complications ● Outcome measured indirectly: Number of dressings/week, wound area remaining, healing scores, and reduction in histologically documented inflammation
● The study design	Experimental and observational studies: *(see Box 1.4)*	● Randomized controlled trials ● Experimental studies without randomization ● Cohort studies with concurrent controls

See case study 3 for a related review

Free form question: Do home visits improve the health of elderly people?

Structured question

● The population	Elderly people in various age groups:	● Young-old ● Middle age-old ● Old-old
● The interventions	Home visits: *versus* Comparator:	● Intensive assessments ● Frequent assessments *versus* ● Usual care
● The outcomes	Various measures to quantify health and health resource use:	● Critical outcome measured directly: Mortality ● Critical outcome measured directly: Functional status ● Important outcome measured directly: Nursing home admissions
● The study design	Experimental studies: *(see Box 1.4)*	● Randomized controlled trials ● Experimental studies without randomization

See Box 4.5 for a related meta-analysis

Free form question: Do antibiotics improve children's outcome in otitis media?

Structured question

● The population	Children with otitis media:	● Various age groups
● The interventions	Antibiotics: *versus*	● Different preparations *versus*
	Comparator:	● Placebo or no treatment
● The outcomes	Various measures to quantify health:	● Critical outcome measured directly: Perforation
		● Important outcome measured directly: Pain
		● Important outcome measured directly: Adverse effects
● The study design	Experimental studies: (*see Box 1.4*)	● Randomized controlled trials
		● Experimental studies without randomization

See Boxes 5.2 and 5.3 for a related review

An example question about clinical and cost-effectiveness

Free form question: To what extent is the risk of post-operative infection reduced by antimicrobial prophylaxis in patients undergoing hip replacement and is it worth the costs?

Structured question

● The population	Patients undergoing hip replacement:	● Various types of procedures
● The interventions	Antimicrobial prophylaxis: *versus*	● Various types of antibiotics *versus*
	Comparator:	● Placebo
		● No antibiotics
● The outcomes	Clinical:	● Post-operative infection
	Economic:	● Cost per infection prevented
● The study design	Clinical:	● Experimental studies (*see Box 1.4*)
	Economic:	● Cost-effectiveness analyses

See Box 3.4 for a related review

An example question about comparing beneficial and harmful outcomes

Free form question: Which rennin-system inhibitor is better in treating hypertension and is it worth the costs?

Structured question

● The population	Patients with hypertension:	● Various co-morbidities
● The interventions	Angiotensin receptor blockers: *versus*	● Various types *versus*

	Angiotensin converting enzyme inhibitors: (avoiding comparison with placebo)	• Various types
• The outcomes	Clinical:	• Critical beneficial outcome measured directly: Mortality and major cardiovascular events • Important beneficial outcome measured indirectly: Renal failure measured by serum creatinine • Important beneficial outcome measured directly: Successful monotherapy • Important adverse outcomes measured directly: Cough and withdrawals
• The study design	Mixture of designs: (*see Box 1.4*)	• Experimental studies for beneficial effects • Observational studies for adverse effects

See Boxes C7.1 and C8.1 for a related review

1.3 Variations in study designs

Let us turn our attention to *study design*, the fourth component of a review question (Box 1.1). For a given set of *populations*, *interventions* and *outcomes*, reviews will provide summaries of existing studies that used different research *designs* (Box 1.2). Why is *design* so important? *Design* of a study determines the validity of the observed effects, i.e. our confidence that the results of a study are likely to approximate to the 'truth' for the participants or patients studied depends on the soundness of its *design*. In this way *design* serves as a marker of study quality. Its importance cannot be emphasized enough. Ultimately the strength of a review's inferences depends on the integrity of the *designs* of the available studies.

Some reviewers consider certain *study designs* to be superior because they feel that the *design* has an inherent value in itself. For example, they may focus exclusively on randomized studies when conducting reviews. Such a view ignores the fact that addressing different types of questions may require the use of different *study designs*. As an example, a question about accuracy of a test would require a *study design* that prospectively (without randomization) recruits all eligible patients, employs the *test* and the *reference standard* investigation to confirm or refute the presence of disease, and determines the accuracy with which the test correctly identifies disease (as in Case study 4). Assessment of long-term or rare *outcomes*, particularly when examining the safety of *interventions* (as in Case study 2), would be more suited to an observational *design*, not an experimental study. For example, cohort and case-control studies, not randomized trials, would evaluate the effect of *exposure* to benzodiazepines in pregnancy on rare malformations in the newborn baby (Box 5.2).

Valid results are said to be unbiased. **Bias** either exaggerates or underestimates the 'true' effect of an *intervention* or *exposure*.

The **quality** of a study depends on the degree to which its design, conduct and analysis minimizes **biases**.

Even for questions concerning effectiveness of *interventions*, where randomized trials are generally preferred, it might be difficult to justify a restriction to using randomized studies only. This may be particularly true when such studies are unethical. Sometimes there is just a dearth of randomized studies. For example, in the review on antimicrobials for chronic wounds (Case study 3), despite a comprehensive search, only four clearly randomized studies could be found, so other *designs* had to be included. On the other hand, in Case study 2, where the review considered safety of water fluoridation, no randomized studies had been published, so it became necessary to consider various other *designs*. Effects of educational interventions are often studied using a range of *designs* (Case study 6). For evaluation of harmful *outcomes* that are rare, observational design is frequently included in reviews (Case study 8). Sometimes a review may consider a number of separate but related questions. For example, if a review is to include an assessment of efficiency in addition to effectiveness, then *study designs* for economic evaluation will also be required (Box 1.3). Thus, it might be necessary to consider different *designs* simultaneously in some review questions. This multiplicity of *designs* has implications for study quality assessment (Step 3) and synthesis (Step 4).

Insistence on randomized studies, ignoring other types of evidence, might paralyse reviewers as such reviews might never find any studies. Often because of ethical or technical reasons the best possible evidence can only be obtained from observational studies. When faced with having to make decisions for practice, using the best available evidence is likely to be better than not using any evidence at all. We will need to explore the nature of our questions (effectiveness, aetiology, efficiency, accuracy, prognosis, etc) and the different ways of addressing the specific issues before us, i.e. *populations*, *interventions* and *outcomes*. Then we should select the *study designs* that are likely to provide the most valid answers and develop a hierarchy of *study designs* suitable for our review. This approach will help us define inclusion and exclusion criteria for selecting studies of a minimum acceptable quality (Step 2). Once studies have been included in a review, a detailed assessment of their quality (Step 3) and results (Step 4) will be required to gauge the strength of the evidence (Step 5).

Each question type has a *design* hierarchy of its own. In this section of the book we focus mainly on questions relating to health effects of *interventions* and *exposures*. These questions usually focus on how one *intervention* or *exposure* compares with another. A hierarchy of *designs* for studies addressing such issues is shown in Box 1.4. The most sound *study design* in this context is one that randomly allocates (concealing the assignment code) participants from a relevant *population* to the alternative *interventions* of interest. This *design* serves to remove selection

Effectiveness is the extent to which an *intervention* (therapy, prevention, diagnosis, screening, education, social care, etc.) produces beneficial *outcomes* under ordinary day-to-day circumstances.

Efficiency (cost-effectiveness) is the extent to which the balance between input (costs) and output (*outcomes*) of *interventions* represents value for money.

Box 1.4 A hierarchy of *study designs* for questions about effectiveness of healthcare interventions

Description of the *design*

Experimental study

A comparative study* in which the use of different interventions among participants is allocated by the researcher.

- **Randomized controlled trial (with concealed allocation)**
  Random allocation of participants to an intervention and a control (e.g. placebo or usual care) group, with follow-up to examine differences in outcomes between the two groups. Randomization (with concealment of allocation sequence from caregivers) avoids bias because both known and unknown determinants of outcome, apart from the intervention, are usually equally distributed between the two groups of participants.

- **Experimental study without randomization** (sometimes erroneously called quasi-experimental or quasi-randomized or pseudo-randomized studies)
  A study in which the allocation of participants to different interventions is managed by the researcher but the method of allocation falls short of genuine randomization, e.g. alternate or even–odd allocation. Such methods fail to conceal the allocation sequence from caregivers.

Observational study with control group

A comparative study* in which the use of different interventions among participants is not allocated by the researcher (it is merely observed).

- **Cohort study**
  Follow-up of participants who receive an intervention (that is not allocated by the researcher) to examine the difference in outcomes compared to a control group, e.g. participants receiving no care.
- **Case–control studies**
  Comparison of intervention rates between participants with the outcome (cases) and those without the outcome (controls).

Observational study without control groups

- **Cross-sectional study**
  Examination of the relationship between outcomes and other variables of interest (including interventions) as they exist in a relevant population at one particular time.
- **Before-and-after study**
  Comparison of outcomes in study participants before and after an intervention.
- **Case series**
  Description of a number of cases of an intervention and their outcomes.

Case reports

- Pathophysiological studies or bench research
- Expert opinion or consensus

A comparative study assesses the effect of an intervention using comparison groups. See Box 1.1 for an example flow chart of such a study

bias and when conducted well, such studies rank at the top of the *study design* hierarchy for effectiveness evidence. Studies where the allocation of participants or patients falls short of genuine randomization and allocation concealment have an inherent risk of bias, and in the evaluation of strength of evidence they are assigned a low level initially (Step 5). Reviewers' inability to recognize valid *designs* can have serious implications for evidence-based practice. For example, relying on expert opinion when reviewing literature could mislead practice recommendations, e.g. erroneously withholding thrombolytic therapy in myocardial infarction. In this field experts have lagged a decade behind strong evidence of effect of this intervention on mortality (*JAMA* 1992; **268**: 240-8).

As indicated above, for many reviews experimental studies will not exist (Case study 2) or they might be scarce (Case study 3). Hence, reviews may have to be conducted using studies of an inferior *design* or using studies with a mixture of *designs*. If our review has several *study designs*, it would be prudent to carefully plan quality assessments (Step 3), stratify study synthesis by *design* and quality (Step 4) and interpret findings cautiously (Step 5). Reviewers who do not take a cautious approach to the *design* issue can easily produce erroneous conclusions, to the detriment of patients. For example, initial recommendations that postmenopausal women use hormone replacement therapy to reduce cardiovascular risk came from observational studies with inconsistent results. Recognition of the limitations of the evidence would have tempered the recommendations, avoiding the need to reverse recommendations when randomized evidence showed that hormone replacement therapy fails to reduce cardiovascular risk and may even increase it (*Ann Intern Med* 2002; **137**: 273-84).

1.4 Modification of questions during a review

It is important that review questions are formulated *a priori*, that is, before the review work is actually commenced. Otherwise the review process may be unduly driven by presuming particular findings. In order to get the questions correct at the beginning, it may be worth involving experienced reviewers and practitioners in the process. This is just one of several reasons why it is considered unwise to prepare a review alone.

Questions will initially be developed without detailed knowledge of much of the relevant literature. Therefore, we should not be surprised if it becomes evident during the review that some questions need to be modified in light of the accumulated research. The commandment 'thou shall pose questions for a review *a priori*' should not be applied too rigidly. We should allow exploration of unexpected issues into the review process; as a greater understanding of the problem is developed during the course of the review, it would be foolish not to do so. If the ongoing work identifies a need for answering questions which had not been foreseen, it would be quite reasonable to raise new questions or to modify existing questions. Such modifications are justifiable if they are based on the realization of alternative ways of defining the *populations*, *interventions*, *outcomes* or *study designs*, which were not considered earlier.

Revision of questions will inevitably have some implications for the review work. The protocol would have to be revised. Literature searches (Step 2), which are usually conducted before questions are refined, may also need refinement and they might have to be run again in the light of the changes to the questions. Study selection criteria will have to be altered. For example, in the review of safety of water fluoridation in Case study 2, the original questions were modified in the light of information gathered about the extent and range of quality of available evidence during the initial part of the review. This led to changes in study selection criteria, which are provided in detail in the published report of the review (www.york.ac.uk/inst/crd/fluorid.htm). Reviewers should not be economical with the truth about question formulation and refinement. It is essential to be explicit about the modifications and indicate which questions were posed *a priori* and which were generated during the review work.

Summary of Step 1: Framing questions for a review

Key points about appraising review articles
- Examine the abstract and the introduction to see if the review is based on predefined questions.
- Examine the methods and other sections to check if questions were modified during the review process.
- Can we be sure that the questions have not been unduly influenced by the knowledge of results of the studies?

Key points about conducting reviews
- The problems to be addressed by the review should be specified in the form of clear, unambiguous questions before beginning the review work.
- Questions should be structured, e.g. in terms of *population*, *interventions*, *outcomes* and *study designs* relevant to the issues being addressed in the review.
- Characteristics of the *populations*, differences in *interventions*, variation in *outcomes* and variety in *study designs* may influence the results of a review. The impact of these factors should be carefully considered at this stage.
- Once the review questions have been set, modifications to the protocol should only be allowed after careful consideration. Sometimes, alternative ways of defining the *populations*,

interventions, outcomes or *study designs* become apparent after commencing the review. In this situation it would be reasonable to alter the original questions, but these modifications should not be driven by the knowledge of results of the studies.

● Step 2: *Identifying relevant literature*

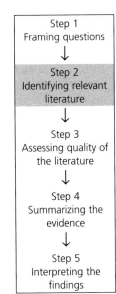

Step 1
Framing questions
↓
Step 2
Identifying relevant literature
↓
Step 3
Assessing quality of the literature
↓
Step 4
Summarizing the evidence
↓
Step 5
Interpreting the findings

Being thorough when identifying the relevant literature is crucial for a systematic review. It is driven by the desire to capture as many relevant studies as possible. In published reviews, literature searches are often summarized too simplistically to allow others to replicate them. A good search can vary between simple and relatively complex, depending on the review topic. Not all searches are beyond the reach of novice reviewers.

A comprehensive literature search includes multistage and iterative processes. First we will need to generate lists of citations from relevant resources (e.g. electronic bibliographic databases, reference lists of known primary and review articles, and relevant journals). Second, we will need to screen these citations for relevance to our review questions with a view to obtaining the full manuscripts of all potentially relevant studies. Third, we will need to sift through these manuscripts to make the final inclusion/exclusion decisions based on explicit study selection criteria. Some of the studies will provide reference lists from which we will find more potentially relevant citations, and the cycle of obtaining manuscripts and examining them for relevance will go one more round. These processes will eventually lead to a set of studies on which the review will be based. In the report of our review, a flowchart of the study identification process will be required (Box 2.1). The basic principles behind the identification of relevant literature covering various aspects of this flowchart are covered in this Step.

2.1 Generating a list of potentially relevant citations

Both the precision and the validity of the findings of reviews are directly related to the comprehensiveness of the literature identification processes. The aim of the initial searches, both electronic and manual, is to generate as comprehensive a list of citations as possible to address the questions being posed in the review. Thus, the search strategy (search terms and the resources to be searched) will depend on the components of the questions. If we have formulated the questions well, we have already made a head start. In practical terms, developing a search strategy may take several iterations, so we should be prepared for the hard work. However, using a systematic approach (similar to the one outlined below) can quickly lead us to a reasonably effective strategy.

The steps involved in electronically generating lists of potentially relevant citations include selection of relevant databases,

Precision of effect in a review refers to its uncertainty. Poor searches may contribute to uncertainty by identifying only a fraction of the available studies, which leads to wide confidence intervals around the summary effects. **Imprecision** refers to uncertainty arising due to play of chance, but not due to **bias**.

Validity of a review refers to the methods used to minimize **bias**. **Bias** will either exaggerate or underestimate the 'true' effect being sought in a review. Poor searches contribute to **bias** as they may preferentially identify studies with particularly positive or particularly negative effects.

Box 2.1 A flowchart describing the process of identifying relevant literature

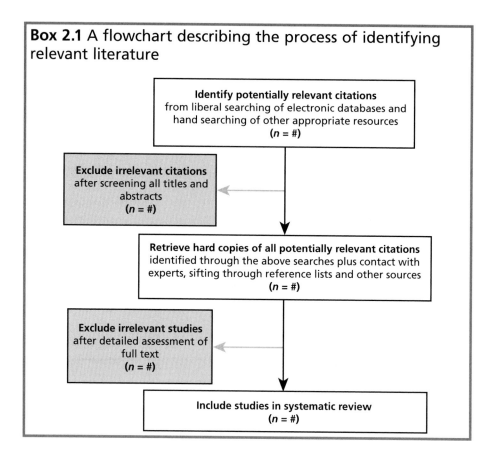

Identify potentially relevant citations
from liberal searching of electronic databases and
hand searching of other appropriate resources
(*n* = #)

Exclude irrelevant citations
after screening all titles and
abstracts
(*n* = #)

Retrieve hard copies of all potentially relevant citations
identified through the above searches plus contact with
experts, sifting through reference lists and other sources
(*n* = #)

Exclude irrelevant studies
after detailed assessment of
full text
(*n* = #)

Include studies in systematic review
(*n* = #)

formulation of an appropriate combination of search terms and retrieval of citations from the searches. Searches undertaken at the beginning of the review may have to be updated at a later date depending on the length of time taken to complete the review.

2.1.1 Selection of relevant databases to search

There exists no such database that covers all publications from all healthcare journals. Serious reviewers usually search many databases. How should we decide about database coverage? This depends very much on the topic of the review. Why not compare and contrast the types of databases searched in Case study 2 (Box C2.1) with those searched in Case study 3 (Box C3.1): the differences are mainly due to differences in the nature of the review topics. There are many useful databases and we may wish to ask our local librarian or consult one of the guides to databases. Some of the commonly used databases are shown in Box 2.2.

Most reviews would include searches in general databases such as Medline and Embase, which cover many of the same journals. Medline is produced by the US National Library of Medicine and has a North American emphasis. Embase has a greater European

Box 2.2 Important databases of research in healthcare

Selected general databases

MEDLINE (available freely via PubMed at www.ncbi.nlm.nih.gov/PubMed)
Bibliographic records (with and without abstracts) of biomedical literature from 1966 onwards.
EMBASE (www.embase.com)
Records of biomedical literature from 1974 onwards.
Science Citation Index (thomsonreuters.com/products_services/science/science_products/scholarly_research_analysis/research_discovery/web_of_science)
Relevant studies found through electronic or manual searches can be used to identify further relevant citations by electronically locating other citations on the same topic through citation search on Science Citation Index.

Selected databases with a specific focus

PsycInfo (http://psycinfo.apa.org/psycinfo/)
Records of literature on psychology and related behavioural and social sciences from 1967.
CENTRAL (The Cochrane Central Register of Controlled Trials – www.thecochranelibrary.com)
Records of clinical trials in healthcare identified through the work of the Cochrane Collaboration, including large numbers of citations from MEDLINE and EMBASE as well as citations not covered by these databases. In the 3rd issue of the 2009 Cochrane Library there were approximately 500 000 trials in CENTRAL.
CINAHL (Cumulative Index to Nursing and Allied Health Literature – www.cinahl.com)
Records of literature on all aspects of nursing and allied health disciplines.
NHS EED (NHS Economic Evaluation Database – www.crd.york.ac.uk/crdweb)
Structured abstracts of economic evaluations of healthcare interventions identified by regular searching of bibliographic databases, hand searching of key major medical journals.
MIDIRS (www.midirs.org)
A broad reference resource available to obstetricians, midwives and consumers.
Conference Papers Index (http://ca2.csa.com/factsheets/cpi-set-c.php)
Records of conference presentations.
Research Registers (for research in progress)
Guide to selected registers – www.york.ac.uk/inst/crd/htadbase.htm
UK Clinical Research Network: Portfolio Database – http://public.ukcrn.org.uk/search
MetaRegister of Current Controlled Trials – http://controlled-trials.com
www.nci.nih.gov/clinical_trials
SIGLE (System for Information on Grey Literature – www.stneasy.fiz-karlsruhe.de)
Bibliographic database covering European non-conventional (so-called grey) literature in the field of pure and applied natural sciences and other areas.
See Boxes C2.1, C3.2, C5.1 and C6.1 for some other databases searched in the case studies.

emphasis in terms of the journals it covers and has a high pharmacological content. Local medical libraries or professional bodies may provide free access to both Medline and Embase. To complicate matters, there are a number of different commercial software interfaces for electronic databases, e.g. Ovid, Silverplatter, Knowledgefinder, etc. Their mode of searching is flexible and user-friendly, but they are more costly than the PubMed interface to Medline which is freely available on the Internet. The PubMed interface has an additional searching feature via its 'Related Articles' function, which allows capture of additional citations on the basis of their similarity to known relevant citations.

2.1.2 Search term combination for electronic database searches

In simple terms, building a suitable combination of search terms involves combining free text words and controlled terms (MeSH or MeSH-like terms) which represent the various components of the review question.

We should begin by examining the *populations*, *interventions*, *outcomes* and *study designs* relevant to our review, as shown in Box 2.3. For each one of these components we will need to compile a list of words that authors might have used in their studies. We may identify a range of synonyms with spelling variations by examining the relevant studies we already know of. These will provide the free text words for our search. We will also need to compile a list of controlled terms that database indexers might have used when recording the citations. There are many ways to identify relevant MeSH or MeSH-like terms. For example, we may look at the key words suggested for indexing in known relevant studies (frequently found at the end of the abstract) and check how they are actually indexed in the databases we want to search. We need to keep in mind that indexers don't always follow authors' suggestions. Each database has its own thesaurus or index structure and we may want to refer to this for additional MeSH terms. This task is made easier in databases that offer the opportunity to map free text words we have selected to MeSH in their index lists. However we select our search terms, we must ensure that an adequate number of free text words and controlled terms are included to represent each component of the question. This will enhance the sensitivity of our search, increasing our ability to capture a large proportion of the relevant studies.

The next stage is to combine the words and terms we have selected to capture the various components of the question. This is achieved by Boolean logic which commonly uses the operators AND, OR and NOT to create sets of citations from the search terms. For example, combining *coke* OR *cola* will retrieve all citations where either one or both of these terms are found. On the other hand, combining *coke* AND *cola* will only retrieve citations where both of these terms are found. Combining *coke*

MeSH or medical subject headings are controlled terms used in the MEDLINE database to index citations. Other bibliographic databases use MeSH-like terms.

Sensitivity of a search is the proportion of relevant studies identified by a search strategy expressed as a percentage of all relevant studies on a given topic. It is a measure of the comprehensiveness of a search method. *Do not confuse with sensitivity of a test.*

Boolean logic refers to the logical relationship among search terms.

Boolean operators AND, OR and NOT are used during literature searches to include or exclude certain citations from electronic databases. An example of their use in PubMed is shown below:

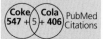

Coke = **552**
Cola = **411**
Coke **AND** Cola = **5**
Coke **OR** Cola = **958**
Coke **NOT** Cola = **547**

Box 2.3 How to develop a search term combination for searching electronic bibliographic databases

An example of a search term combination for Ovid MEDLINE database

Free form question: In women undergoing surgical termination of pregnancy, does antibiotic prophylaxis reduce the risk of post-operative infection?

Structured question (not all components may be needed for searching)

- The population — Pregnant women undergoing surgical abortion
- The interventions — • Antibiotics used as prophylaxis
  - • Comparator: placebo or no intervention (not used in search term combination)
- The outcome — Post-operative infection
- The study design — Experimental studies (not used in search term combination)

Question components and relevant search terms	Type of terms		Boolean operator
	Free	MeSH	
The population: Pregnant women undergoing surgical abortion			
1 (terminat$ adj3 pregnan$).tw	X		
2 (unwant$ adj3 pregnan$).tw	X		
3 abortion$.tw	X		OR (captures *population*)
4 exp abortion induced/		X	
5 exp pregnancy unwanted/		X	
6 or/1–5			
The interventions: Antibiotics used as prophylaxis			
7 exp infection control/		X	
8 exp anti-infective agents/		X	
9 exp antibiotics/		X	OR (captures *interventions*)
10 antibiotic$.tw	X		
11 (antibiotic adj3 prophyla$).tw	X		
12 (antimicrobial$ or anti-microbial$).tw	X		
13 or/7–12			
The outcome: Post-operative infection			
14 exp bacterial infections/		X	
15 exp postoperative complications/		X	
16 sepsis/		X	
17 exp abortion septic/		X	
18 exp endometritis/		X	
19 exp adnexitis/		X	
20 (postoperative adj3 (infect$ or contaminat$ or complicat$ or pyrexi$)).tw	X		OR (captures *outcome*)

Question components and relevant search terms	Type of terms		Boolean operator
	Free	MeSH	
21 (sepsis or septic).tw	x		
22 (bacteria$ adj3 (contaminat$ or infect$)).tw	x		
23 (post-abort$ adj3 (infect$ or complicat$ or contaminat$)).tw	x		
24 endometritis.tw	x		
25 pelvic inflammatory disease.tw	x		
26 (septic adj3 abort$).tw	x		
27 or/14–26			
28 and/6,13,27			AND (combines all components)

Commands and symbols for Ovid Medline

$ Truncation, e.g. pregnan$ will pick up pregnant, pregnancy and pregnancies

adj   Proximity and adjacency searching, e.g. terminat$ adj pregnan$ means that these terms appear next to each other, terminat$ adj3 pregnan$ means that there may be three other words in between them

.tw   Textword search, e.g. abortion$.tw, will search for textwords in title or abstract

/   Medical subject heading (MeSH) search, e.g. abortion induced/, will search for MeSH in indexing terms

exp   Explodes the MeSH, e.g. exp abortion induced/ will search for this MeSH as well as the lower order MeSH terms included under the MeSH abortion induced in tree structure, such as abortion eugenic, abortion legal, abortion therapeutic, pregnancy reduction multifetal

See related selection criteria in Box 2.5
Based on RCOG Clinical Governance Advice No. 3 (www.rcog.org.uk/mainpages. asp?PageID=318)

NOT *cola* will retrieve citations that contain the term *coke* only, thereby excluding all citations with the term *cola*. Needless to say, NOT should be used with great caution. In general, one would use OR to combine all the words and terms capturing a component of the question. This will give a large citation set for each component that we searched for. We can now combine these with AND to produce a set which contains citations relevant to all the various components of the question.

Box 2.3 only shows the search term combinations for the Medline database. Any search term combinations developed for MEDLINE would need to be adapted to the peculiarities of each of the other databases to be searched. This may require professional support. It can be guaranteed that this will not be easy, particularly because different databases use different terms and index structures. But we should not lose sight of our objective, which is to produce a valid answer for the questions raised for the review. There is substantial evidence that limiting the search to only a few databases tends to bias the review. The more broad based our search, the more likely it is that our review will produce a precise and valid answer.

2.1.3 Searching for study designs

One important component of the review question is *study design*, which can be used to improve our search strategy. For example, to identify published and unpublished clinical trials we may search specialist collections such as the Cochrane Central Register of Controlled Trials (CENTRAL) and research registers of ongoing trials (http://controlled-trials.com). These are usually the first databases to be searched in reviews of randomized studies. However, for other *study designs* such collections are rare.

General databases have subject indexing for some study designs but this alone may not be adequate for searching. Therefore search term combinations which capture studies of a particular design (also known as search filters) have been developed by information specialists. It is tempting to search general databases using such *design* filters, e.g. those available on PubMed Clinical Queries (www.ncbi.nlm.nih.gov/corehtml/query/static/clinical.shtml) or on other health technology assessment websites, e.g. www.york.ac.uk/inst/crd/intertasc/. Some filters are designed to perform quick searches to support day-to-day evidence-based practice. They will make our search more precise but inevitably this will be at the expense of sensitivity. This means that a high proportion of citations retrieved by filtered searches will be relevant, but many relevant citations will be missed because they are not indexed in a way that the filter can pick up. This is a major drawback because systematic reviews should be based on searches that are as thorough as possible. There is one exception – for reviews of randomized trials where indexing of *design*-related terms is more reasonable, carefully adapted versions of existing filters for therapy questions may be used (see Case study 3). Case study 5 demonstrates the use of a qualitative research design filter (Box C5.1) and Case study 8 illustrates the use of an observational study design filter to capture literature on adverse effects.

> **Precision of a search** is the proportion of relevant studies identified by a search strategy. This is expressed as a percentage of all studies (relevant and irrelevant) identified by that strategy. It is a measure of the ability of a search to exclude irrelevant studies. *Do not confuse with precision of effect.*

> **Study design filter** employs a search term combination to capture citations of studies of a particular design.

2.1.4 Reference lists and other sources (e.g. journals, grey literature, conference proceedings)

Inaccurate or incomplete indexing of articles and journals in electronic bibliographic databases requires the examination of other sources of citations. Reference lists from identified studies and related reviews provide a rich source of potentially relevant citations. Index Medicus and Excerpta Medica can be manually searched if it is desirable to identify studies prior to the start dates of the electronic databases (as in Case study 2). The latest issues of the key journals may also be searched to identify very recent studies which have not yet been included on the electronic databases or cited by others. It can take some time for studies published in some journals indexed in Medline to finally appear in this database.

Many studies published in technical reports, discussion papers or other formats are not included in major databases and journals, but some of these may be indexed on databases such as SIGLE (System for Information on Grey Literature), the National Technical Information Service (www.ntis.gov), and the British National Bibliography for Report Literature (www.bl.uk/). The libraries of specialist research organizations and professional societies may provide another useful source of this grey literature. Dissertations and theses can also be routes into obtaining otherwise unpublished research and these are recorded in databases such as Dissertation Abstracts and CINAHL (Cumulative Index to Nursing and Allied Health Literature). Conference proceedings can provide information on research in progress as well as completed research. You can access this information through the Index of Scientific and Technical Proceedings, the Conference Papers Index and in the catalogues of large research libraries.

2.1.5 Identifying ongoing research

The most unbiased study retrieval can only be guaranteed in those few areas where prospective comprehensive research registers are maintained. These research registers may provide information on completed or ongoing studies. Box 2.2 shows some electronic resources to search for ongoing studies. Many pharmaceutical companies hold their study results in private databases, which may occasionally be released on request (as in Case study 1).

Bias in study retrieval will either exaggerate or underestimate the 'true' effect being sought in a review. Poor searches contribute to **bias** as they may preferentially identify studies with particularly positive or particularly negative effects.

2.1.6 Searching the internet

This is how research is increasingly being published and accessed. Many of the electronic databases described above are available through the internet. The 'world wide web' can also be used to identify researchers and manufacturers as well as completed and ongoing studies. Given the enormity of the web, any serious attempt to search it would be a major undertaking, with tens of thousands of web pages to browse. A structured approach would have to be developed, e.g. using meta-search engines (e.g. Dogpile – www.dogpile.com, Google – www.google.com, etc.), or search engines with a healthcare focus (e.g. Turning Research Into Practice – www.tripdatabase.com/, Intute – www.intute. ac.uk/, etc.). Sometimes it is much more efficient to look for evidence that already has been pre-selected by experts. The BMJ Group and McMaster University's Health Information Research Unit provide access to current best evidence from research, tailored to one's own healthcare interests, to support evidence-based clinical decisions. Citations (from over 130 premier clinical journals) are pre-rated for quality by research staff, then rated for clinical relevance and interest by at least three members of a worldwide panel of practising physicians. http://plus.mcmaster.ca/EvidenceUpdates/Default.aspx

2.1.7 Seeking professional input

After reading through this section you might feel that literature identification is beyond your current searching skills and you will need professional input. Many professional reviewers receive support from information specialists to carry out their searches. Your local librarian may be able to help – they might be able to direct you to an information service that conducts systematic literature searches. Registering your review with a relevant Review Group of the Cochrane Collaboration might allow you access to professional searches. Many of the Review Groups have developed comprehensive search strategies in their topics and maintain specialized registers.

2.2 Citation retrieval and management

In order to effectively manage the process of literature identification, citations obtained from the searches will have to be imported into a computer program for reference management (e.g. Reference Manager, ProCite, EndNote). Construction of a master citation database for a review will involve collating all the citations from various sources. Built-in functions of the citation management software allow exact and inexact duplicates (where titles, authors or journal names of the same articles are cited or stated in different manners) to be easily detected. Additional functions of the software can add labels or tags to the citations, by creation of user defined fields, allowing for enhanced sorting and documentation of the selection process. Searches of some of the sources (e.g. CENTRAL) may not be importable directly into the master citation database. Citations from these sources will have to be scrutinized and managed using simple word-processing software. In addition, searches of non-electronic sources (e.g. reference lists of known articles) may be managed manually. Eventually many citations will have to be manually entered into the master citation database of the review.

The **Cochrane Collaboration** is an international collaboration that aims to help with informed decision making on healthcare topics by preparing, maintaining and ensuring accessibility of systematic reviews of interventions (www.cochrane.org).

2.3 Selecting relevant studies

The aim of the study selection process is to use the citation lists to identify those articles that definitely address the questions being posed in the review. This is part of the multi-stage process described in Box 2.1. The process consists of defining the study selection criteria, screening the citations to obtain the full reports

Selecting relevant citations
- Develop selection criteria
- Select relevant citations
- Obtain full papers and select those relevant
- Do not use language restrictions

of all studies that are likely to meet the selection criteria, and sifting through these manuscripts to make the final inclusion/exclusion decisions.

2.3.1 Study selection criteria

These should follow on logically from the review question. Box 2.4 shows example sets of selection criteria defined in terms of the *populations, interventions, outcome* and *study designs* of interest. Ultimately, only studies that meet all of the inclusion criteria (and none of the exclusion criteria) will be included in the review. To avoid bias in the selection process, the criteria (both inclusion and exclusion) should be defined *a priori*.

When defining selection criteria, we should ask ourselves:

- Is it sensible to group various *populations* together?
- Is it sensible to combine various *interventions* together?
- What *outcomes* are clinically relevant?
- What *study designs* should be included/excluded?

Often reviewers are led by what is likely to be reported rather than by what is clinically important, but it is preferable to select studies with clinical importance rather than surrogate *outcomes* (Step 1). The decision taken about study selection, whatever it is, will have consequences for the rest of the review. It is up to us as the reviewers to decide on how broad or narrow the selection criteria should be. Criteria that are too broadly defined may make it difficult to synthesize studies; criteria that are too narrowly defined may reduce the applicability of the findings of our review. A balanced approach can enhance the applicability of our findings. For example, using liberal inclusion criteria concerning the *populations* may allow investigation of questions concerning the variation in effects among different *population* subgroups (see Box 4.5).

Ideally studies of the most robust *design* should be included. However, practically, the criteria concerning *study design* may be influenced by knowing the type and amount of available literature to some extent after initiating the review. If the selection criteria are modified in the light of the information gathered from the initial searches, the modifications should be justified and explicitly reported. When studies of robust *designs* have not been carried out (Case study 2) or if they are scarce (Case study 3), the inclusion criterion specifying the *study design* may have to consider studies of methodologically poorer quality. This approach may be used in reviews where the goal is to summarize the currently available evidence for decision making, as in Case studies 2, 3 and 6. If a review has several *study designs*, this will have implications on study quality assessments (Step 3), study synthesis (Step 4) and interpretation of findings (which should be cautious) based mainly on methodologically superior studies (Step 5).

Box 2.4 Some examples of study selection criteria

Free form question: In women undergoing surgical termination of pregnancy, does antibiotic prophylaxis reduce the risk of post-operative infection? (*see structured question in Box 2.3*)

Question component	Inclusion criteria	Exclusion criteria
● The population	Pregnant women undergoing surgical abortion	Other operations
● The interventions	Antibiotics compared to placebo or no prophylaxis; comparison of different antibiotics	Lack of comparison
● The outcome	Post-operative infection confirmed by appropriate microbiological techniques	Infection not confirmed
● The study design	Experimental studies	Observational studies

Free form question: Is it safe to provide population-wide drinking water fluoridation to prevent caries?

Question component	Inclusion criteria	Exclusion criteria
● The population	Population receiving drinking water sourced through a public water supply	Unsourced water supply
● The interventions	Fluoridation of drinking water, naturally occurring or artificially added, compared to non-fluoridated water	Lack of comparison
● The outcome	Cancer, bone fractures and fluorosis	Other outcomes
● The study design	– Experimental studies – Observational studies (cohort, case-control, cross-sectional, and before-and-after)	– Case series – Case reports

See Case study 2 for a related review

Free form question: Which of the many available antimicrobial products improve healing in patients with chronic wounds? (*see structured question in Box 1.3*)

Question component	Inclusion criteria	Exclusion criteria
● The population	Adults with chronic wounds	Other wounds
● The interventions	Systemic and topical antimicrobial preparations compared to placebo or no antimicrobial; comparison of different antibiotics	Lack of comparison

Question component	Inclusion criteria	Exclusion criteria
• The outcome	Wound healing	Wound healing not assessed
• The study design	– Randomized controlled trials – Experimental studies without randomization – Cohort studies with concurrent controls	– Studies with historical controls – Case control studies

See Case study 3 for a related review

See Box 1.4 for a brief description of various study designs

2.3.2 Screening of citations

Initially, the selection criteria should be applied liberally to the citation lists generated from searching relevant literature sources. Citations often contain only limited information, so any titles (and abstracts) which seem potentially relevant should provisionally be included for consideration on the basis of the full text articles. However, many citations will clearly be irrelevant and these can be excluded at this stage. Two reviewers should carry out citation screening independently and the full manuscripts of all citations considered relevant by any of the reviewers should be obtained. The yield of this process will vary from one review to another.

2.3.3 Obtaining full manuscripts

From a visit to our nearest medical library we will be able to find out the lists and dates of journals that we can obtain locally. However, first it is worth checking on the internet for freely available journals (www.freemedicaljournals.com) and then download the papers electronically. Your institution or library may also subscribe to electronic journals not freely available. In this way, many recent publications may be quickly obtained. The next Step will be to obtain articles not available through our library or on the internet. This could be time consuming and help from the local librarian or from a librarian at a professional body will be invaluable. On occasion it may be necessary to write to the authors directly to obtain the papers.

2.3.4 Study selection

The final inclusion/exclusion decisions should be made after examining the full texts of all the potentially relevant citations. We should carefully assess the information contained in these to see whether the criteria have been met or not. Many of the doubtful citations initially included may be confidently excluded at this stage. It will be useful to construct a list of excluded studies at this point, detailing the reason for each exclusion. This will not take much time and providing this list as part of our review increases the quality of our report. When submitting a manuscript of a review for publication in a printed journal, it may not be possible to include this section due to restrictions on space. However, these details can be provided in an electronic version of the journal or they could be made available from our offices on request.

Two independent reviewers should undertake assessments of citations and manuscripts for selection because even when explicit inclusion criteria are prespecified, the decisions concerning inclusion/exclusion can be relatively subjective. For example, when applying the *study design* criteria for selection, reviewers may disagree about including or excluding a study due to unclear reporting in the paper. The selection criteria can be initially piloted in a subset of studies where duplicate assessments allow reviewers to assess whether they can be applied in a consistent fashion. If the agreement between the reviewers is poor in the pilot phase, revision of the selection criteria may be required. Once these issues have been clarified, any subsequent disagreements are usually simple oversights, which are easily resolved by consensus. Occasionally arbitration by a third reviewer may be required. Beware of reviews which have only one author; it is likely that errors will have been made in selecting studies.

2.3.5 Selecting studies with duplicate publication

Reviewers often encounter multiple publications of the same study. Sometimes these will be exact duplications, but at other times they might be serial publications with the more recent papers reporting increasing numbers of participants or lengths of follow-up. Inclusion of duplicated data would inevitably bias the data synthesis in the review, particularly because studies with more positive results are more likely to be duplicated. However, the examination of multiple reports of the same study may provide useful information about its quality and other characteristics not captured by a single report. Therefore, all such reports should be examined. However, the data should only be counted once using the largest, most complete report with the longest follow-up.

2.4 Publication and related biases

Identification of all the relevant studies depends on their accessibility. Some studies may be less accessible due to:

- a lack of statistical significance in their results
- the type and language of their reports
- the timing of their publication
- their indexing in databases.

Studies in which *interventions* are not found to be effective, are less likely to be published or they are published in less accessible formats. Publication bias may also involve studies that report certain positive effects that go against strong prevailing beliefs.

Publication bias is said to arise when the likelihood of publication of studies and thus their accessibility to reviewers is related to the significance of their results regardless of their quality.

Systematic reviews that fail to identify such studies will inevitably exaggerate or underestimate the effect of an *intervention* and this is when publication bias arises. Thus the use of a systematic approach to track down less accessible studies is crucial for avoiding bias in systematic reviews. Hopefully in the future, with prospective registration of primary studies, there will be less concern about overlooking studies. Until this happens, it will be necessary to search hard to protect reviews against publication bias. In Step 4 we see how the risk of publication and related biases can be investigated in a review using a funnel plot analysis (Box 4.8).

2.4.1 Searching multiple databases

There is evidence that limiting the search to only a few databases tends to bias the review. We need to cast as wide a net as possible to capture as many citations as possible. Case studies 2 and 3 demonstrate the great lengths serious reviewers can go to when searching for citations. Similarly, if our review is to be taken seriously, we will have to search multiple (overlapping) sources of citations.

2.4.2 Language restrictions in study selection

There is no good reason for excluding articles published in languages that we cannot read or understand. There is increasing evidence that studies with positive findings are more likely to be published in English language journals. Studies with negative findings from non-English speaking countries are frequently published in local language journals. Therefore positive studies are more likely to be accessed if searches are limited to the English language, thereby introducing bias. In addition, language restrictions may decrease the precision of the summary effect in our meta-analysis. For these reasons it may be helpful to find some interpretation facilities. If our review is registered with a relevant Cochrane Review Group, there might be help available for dealing with foreign language papers. Otherwise we may have to tackle this issue by obtaining access to translation facilities or by asking other people to extract the necessary data for us. Sorry, but there is no easy way out.

Summary of Step 2: Identifying relevant literature

Key points about appraising review articles
- Examine the methods section to see if the searches appear to be comprehensive:
  - check if search term combinations follow from the question
  - list the resources (e.g. databases) searched to identify primary studies

- have any relevant resources been left out?
- were any restrictions applied by dates, language, etc?
- Were the selection criteria set *a priori*? How reliably were they applied?
- Have analyses been conducted to examine for the risk of publication and related biases? (see Step 4)
- How likely is it that relevant studies might have been missed? And what is the potential impact on the conclusions of the review?

Key points about conducting reviews

- The search for studies should be extensive and the selection process should minimize bias.
- The search term combination should follow from the question and it should be designed to cast a wide net for capturing as many potentially relevant citations as possible. Multiple resources (both computerized and printed) should be searched. Searches undertaken at the beginning may have to be updated towards the end of the review, depending on the length of time taken to review.
- A systematic approach to citation management should be used to manage the review efficiently.
- Study selection criteria should flow directly from the review questions; they should be set *a priori* and should be piloted to check that they can be reliably applied.
- When sifting through the citations, selection criteria should be applied liberally to retrieve full manuscripts of all potentially relevant citations.
- Final inclusion/exclusion decisions should be made after examination of the full manuscripts. Reasons for inclusion and exclusion should be recorded.
- Language restriction should not be applied in searching or in study selection.
- Duplicate independent assessments of citations and manuscripts should be performed to reduce the risk of errors of judgement in the study selection.
- If feasible, an analysis should be undertaken to explore for the risk of publication and related biases (see Step 4).

● Step 3: *Assessing the quality of the literature*

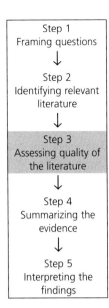

Step 1
Framing questions
↓
Step 2
Identifying relevant literature
↓
Step 3
Assessing quality of the literature
↓
Step 4
Summarizing the evidence
↓
Step 5
Interpreting the findings

It cannot be emphasized enough that the quality of the studies included in a systematic review is the 'Achilles' heel' behind its conclusions. Therefore we should consider study quality at every Step in a review. The quality of a study may be defined as the degree to which it employs measures to minimize bias and error in its *design*, conduct and analysis. We have briefly considered the importance of *study design* as a general marker of study quality when framing questions (Step 1) and selecting studies (Step 2). This approach helps to crudely define the weakest acceptable *study design*, thereby guaranteeing a minimum level of quality.

Once studies of a minimum acceptable quality (based on *design*) have been selected, an in-depth critical appraisal will allow us to assess the quality of the evidence in a more refined way. Step 3 explains how to develop and use checklists for detailed assessments of selected studies for their quality. These refined and detailed quality assessments will be used later in evidence synthesis (Step 4) and interpretation (Step 5). In this way, the checklists will help judge the strength of the evidence collated in a review. In this Step we will focus on quality assessment of studies on effectiveness of *interventions*. The case studies section of this book gives details of quality assessment of studies on safety of *interventions* (Case study 2), accuracy of *tests* (Case study 4), qualitative research (Case study 5), educational effectiveness (Case study 6) and adverse effects of drugs (Case study 8).

3.1 Development of study quality assessment checklists

Quality assessment will usually be based on an appraisal of individual aspects of a study's *design*, conduct and analysis (often called quality items) – evidence of deficiencies may raise the possibility of bias. We can find quality items in one of the many published guides on critical appraisal of healthcare literature (see users' guides to evidence-based practice at www.cche.net/usersguides/main.asp). These guides are usually written for supporting evidence-based practice and provide advice on appraisal of individual studies according to the nature of the clinical query, which we delineate when framing our question (Step 1). The items in these guides can be used as a basis for developing a checklist to perform an in-depth appraisal of the quality of each study included in a review.

There are many published quality assessment checklists for use in systematic reviews; but beware, most have not been developed with scientific rigour. A whole range of quality items is emphasized

Bias either exaggerates or underestimates the 'true' effect of an *intervention* or *exposure*.

Systematic error (or **bias**) leads to effects departing systematically, either lower or higher, from the 'true' effect.

Random error is due to the play of chance and leads to effects being imprecise (wide confidence intervals).

Box 3.1 Study quality assessment in a systematic review

1) Define the question and the selection criteria:

- Consider the nature of the questions being posed
- Consider the types of relevant *study designs*
- Determine a quality threshold (*study design* threshold) which defines the weakest acceptable *design* for selection (Step 2)

2) Develop or select a quality checklist

Identify a suitable existing checklist for your review topic. If one does not exist, develop a new quality checklist considering relevant quality items grouped as follows:

- Generic items related to relevant *study designs* depending on the nature of the review question (usually obtained from published critical appraisal guides or existing quality checklists)
- Specific items related to the *populations, interventions* and *outcomes* of the review question

3) Examine the reliability of checklist use:

- Assess the reliability of the checklist in a pilot phase before applying it to all the selected studies

4) Incorporate the quality assessments into the systematic review

We may use the quality assessment for all or some of the following:

- To describe the quality of studies included in a review
- To explore quality differences as an explanation for the variation in effects from study to study (Step 4)
- To make decisions regarding pooling the effects observed in included studies (Step 4)
- To aid in determining the strength of inferences (Step 5)
- To make recommendations about how future studies could be performed better

in the various checklists but some items may not be related to bias. By assigning numerical values to items, some checklists create a scale in an attempt to provide an overall quantitative quality score for each study. Many checklists neatly classify studies into low or high quality subgroups based on their compliance with the quality items. If we took a leap of faith and randomly selected one of these published quality checklists for our review, we might find ourselves in trouble. On closer examination we might find that not all items in the checklist were relevant to our review, and some relevant items were not part of the checklist. For instance, blind *outcome* assessment is emphasized in most checklists. Blinding might be of marginal importance for an unambiguous *outcome* such as mortality, but it is fundamental in the assessment of subjective *outcomes* such as pain. The numerical values assigned to the items for scoring quality may not be suitable for every review; the same is true of the arbitrariness in the criteria recommended for the low–high dichotomy. It is even possible that variation in the choice of checklist might produce different quality assessments for the same studies. Getting worried? Who would not.

With this background, it should be clear that the published guides on critical appraisal of studies for evidence-based practice or on study quality assessment for systematic reviews are mostly of a generic nature. Ultimately, it is our responsibility to adapt them to our review by considering the issues specific to our questions. If we are lucky, existing reviews on the same topic may have already developed a suitable quality checklist. In this situation re-invention would be pointless and using an existing checklist would also enhance comparability with other reviews on our topic. On the other hand, if there are no suitable existing checklists, we will have to develop one. We will need to identify the individual items for assessing quality carefully and judiciously. How can we recognize which items are important for our review? Studies relevant to the review question may be susceptible to specific biases related to the way in which they are conducted and the data they analysed. Therefore, we will have to be prepared to modify a relevant generic quality checklist, including appropriate additional items and deleting irrelevant ones. Following the approach shown in Box 3.1, the examples in Boxes 3.3 and 3.4, and the demonstrations in the case studies, we should be able to develop a reasonable quality assessment checklist for our review.

3.1.1 Key biases in research addressed by generic quality assessment items

There are many generic biases that reviewers need to consider when developing quality assessment checklists. Bias has been defined as a tendency in research to produce results that depart systematically from the 'true' results. There are several types of biases. Here we shall consider four key biases which impact on the (internal) validity of a study. These are selection bias, performance bias, measurement bias and attrition bias (Box 3.2). Ideally, researchers should try to avoid these biases altogether in primary studies, but we know that they don't. Therefore a very good understanding of these issues must be developed in order to be able to discover biases during study quality assessment in our review. Our efforts may be made difficult or even impossible due to the poverty of reporting in some studies.

A simple study design for an effectiveness study is shown in Box 3.2. An important requirement for valid results in these studies is that the comparison groups should be similar at the beginning. This is because when there is imbalance of relevant prognostic features between groups, it becomes difficult for differences in outcomes to be confidently attributed to the intervention. Technically speaking, this is due to confounding. It is at the time of allocating participants to groups that selection bias arises and it is important to check if appropriate measures were designed and implemented to prevent or minimize it. Experimental studies

Confounding is a situation in comparative studies where the effect of an *intervention* on an *outcome* is distorted due to the association of the *population* and the *outcome* with another factor, which can prevent or cause the *outcome* independent of the *intervention*.

The (internal) **validity** of a study refers to the degree which its results are likely to be free of **bias**.

Bias either exaggerates or underestimates the 'true' effect of an *intervention* or *exposure*.

using random allocation of participants (with concealment of allocation sequence) produce comparison groups that are expected to be balanced for known, unknown and unmeasured prognostic variables. This is the main reason why there has been an emphasis in reviews to focus on randomized trials.

Following the allocation of participants to groups, performance bias may arise due to unintended *interventions* or co-interventions (e.g. other treatments which are not part of the research). We need to assess if the care plans were standardized and if the researchers and the participants were kept blind to the group allocation. We also need to examine if there was a risk of measurement bias, particularly if the *outcomes* assessed were subjective, and if the participants and researchers involved in ascertaining the *outcomes* were not blind to group allocation. In this way blinding is important for preventing both performance and measurement bias.

For preventing attrition bias, an intention-to-treat (ITT) analysis is needed, and it requires data for all patients. Participants' outcomes are analysed according to their initial group allocation, regardless of whether they fully complied with the intervention, changed their intervention group during the study or dropped out of the study before its completion. If the selected studies do not perform their analysis in this way, we may be able to do the calculation ourselves, provided a complete description (numbers and reasons) of the withdrawals is available, including information on both the people who dropped out and those lost to follow-up. If participants withdraw from the study and their *outcome* is unknown, there is no satisfactory way to perform the analysis. The options available include carrying forward the last *outcome* assessment or imputing the best or worst *outcome* for the missing observations in a sensitivity analysis. Thus, if too many participants are lost to follow-up, the analysis may produce biased effects.

In an **intention-to-treat (ITT) analysis**, subjects are analysed according to their initial group allocation, regardless of whether they fully complied with the intervention, changed their intervention group after initial allocation or left the study early.

Withdrawals are participants or patients who do not fully comply with the intervention, cross over and receive an alternative intervention, choose to drop out or are lost to follow-up. **Intention-to-treat** analysis with an appropriate **sensitivity analysis** is required to deal with withdrawals.

Box 3.2 Key biases and their relationship to the design and the quality of a study

A study design to assess the effectiveness of interventions

Simple description

A study that allocates (with or without randomization) subjects from a relevant population to alternative interventions and follows them up to determine the effectiveness with which interventions improve the outcome.

Study flow chart with key biases

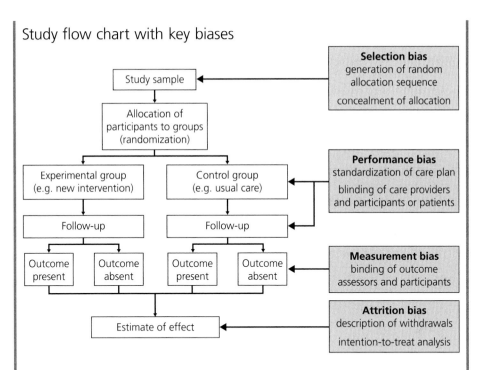

Key biases and their implications for study quality assessment

Type of bias	Relevant generic quality items
Selection bias Systematic differences between comparison groups in prognosis or responsiveness to treatment.	• Generation of random sequence for allocating (large number of) participants to groups • Concealment of allocation from care providers and participants (this can be done in unblinded studies)
Performance bias Systematic differences in care provided apart from the intervention being evaluated.	• Standardization of care protocol • Blinding of clinicians and participants
Measurement bias Systematic differences between comparison groups in how outcomes are ascertained.	• Blinding of participants and outcome assessors
Attrition bias Systematic differences between comparison groups in withdrawals from the study.	• Intention-to-treat analysis (or a complete description of withdrawals to allow such an analysis)

See Box 3.4 for generic quality items based on these biases

Box 3.3 shows how key generic biases can be considered along with biases arising from issues specific to a review concerning the effectiveness of a treatment for infertility. In this example, good quality research requires that couples have a complete set of investigations for infertility before the *interventions* are provided, and that they are followed up for long enough to allow detection of pregnancy. In this way it would be possible to assess if the treatment led to pregnancies more often than the control without the biasing influences of poor diagnostic work-up for infertility and inadequate length of follow-up. These issues are considered along with the generic key biases to produce a checklist for study quality assessment (see Boxes 3.3 and 3.5).

As indicated earlier, the biases related to selection, performance, measurement and attrition are some of the key biases, and they pertain mainly to questions about effectiveness. If our question is about accuracy of tests (Case study 4) or cost-effectiveness (Box 3.4) or some other aspect of healthcare, we will have to consider the biases relevant to these research types for our quality checklist.

Sensitivity analysis involves repetition of an analysis under different assumptions to examine the impact of these assumptions on the results. In a primary study where there are **withdrawals**, a sensitivity analysis may involve repeating the analysis, imputing the best or worst outcome for the missing observations or carrying forward the last outcome assessment.

Box 3.3 Example of developing a study quality assessment checklist in an effectiveness review

1) Define the clinical question and the selection criteria

Free form question: Among infertile couples with subfertility due to a male factor, does anti-oestrogen treatment increase pregnancy rates? (*see structured question in Box 3.5*)

2) Define the selection criteria

- Nature of question   Assessment of clinical effectiveness
- Study design   Comparative studies (see Box 1.4)
- Study design threshold   Inclusion criterion: experimental studies
       Exclusion criterion: observational studies

3) Develop the study quality checklist

a) Generic quality items for the checklist (see *Box 3.4*)

Generation of a random sequence for allocating the patients to the interventions

- Adequate
  - computer-generated random numbers or random number tables
- Inadequate
  - use of alternation, case record numbers, birth dates or week days
- Unclear or unstated

Concealment of allocation

- Adequate
  - centralized real-time or pharmacy-controlled randomization in unblinded studies, or serially numbered identical containers in blinded studies

- other approaches with robust methods to prevent foreknowledge of the allocation sequence to clinicians and patients
- Inadequate
  - use of alternation, case record numbers, birth dates or week days, open random numbers lists, or serially numbered envelopes (even sealed opaque envelopes can be subject to manipulation)
- Unclear or unstated

Blinding
- Adequate
  - care provider and study patients
- Inadequate
  - care provider or study patients
- Unclear or unstated

Description of withdrawals (to allow an intention-to-treat [ITT] analysis)
- Adequate
  - inclusion of all those who dropped out/were lost to follow-up in the analysis
  - numbers *and* reasons provided for each group
  - description allows analysis following the ITT principle
- Inadequate
  - only numbers (*not* reasons) provided for each group
  - description does not allow an analysis following the ITT principle
- Unclear or unstated

b) Specific quality items related to the clinical features of the review question

The population	Complete diagnostic work-up for infertility
The interventions	No relevant items
The outcome	One year follow-up duration to detect pregnancy

4) Incorporate the quality assessments into the review
Some examples of the above quality assessment are as follows:
- To describe the quality of studies included in the review (*see Box 3.5*)
- To aid in determining the strength of inferences (*see Box 4.7*)

3.2 Study quality assessments in reviews with a mixture of *designs*

In the past there has been a strong emphasis for reviews to focus on a single *study design* of the highest quality, i.e. randomized controlled trials (Box 1.4). However, reviewers soon realized that for many important questions, studies of high quality *designs* were often not available (Case study 2) or they were scarce (Case study 3). This is either because no one undertook such studies in the past or if they did try, it was not practicable or ethical to conduct them. When there is a dearth of studies with a high quality *design*, it is not uncommon for reviews to include a mixture of *designs* to summarize the available evidence. This approach carries problems

Box 3.4 Example of developing a study quality assessment checklist in a review with multiple questions

1) Define the question and the selection criteria

Free form question: To what extent is the risk of post-operative infection reduced by antimicrobial prophylaxis, in patients undergoing hip replacement and is it worth the costs? (*see structured question in Box 1.3*)

- Nature of question   Assessment of clinical effectiveness
  Assessment of cost-effectiveness (or efficiency)
    - cost-effectiveness can be assessed by (a) review of all available full economic evaluations, (b) a review of effectiveness studies in conjunction with any available cost sources, and (c) a secondary economic evaluation using the evidence from the effectiveness review to build an economic decision model. In this example, we consider quality assessment for option (a).
- Study design   Effectiveness: Experimental studies
  Cost-effectiveness: Full economic evaluations
- Study design threshold   Effectiveness: (see Box 1.4)
    - inclusion criterion: Experimental studies
    - exclusion criterion: Observational studies
  Cost-effectiveness: (*see glossary*)
    - inclusion criterion: Cost-effectiveness analyses
    - exclusion criterion: Partial economic evaluations

2) Develop the study quality checklist

Some generic quality items for checklists

- Clinical effectiveness review
    - random allocation of patients to groups
    - concealment of allocation sequence
    - pre-specified criteria for eligibility of patients
    - similarity of groups at baseline regarding prognostic factors
    - blinding of care providers, patients and outcome assessors
    - an intention-to-treat analysis
- Cost-effectiveness review
    - a comprehensive description of alternative interventions
    - identification of all important and relevant costs and outcomes for the interventions
    - use of established evidence of clinical effectiveness, i.e. intervention known to improve outcome
    - costs and outcomes measured accurately and valued credibly
    - costs and outcomes adjusted for differential timing
    - an incremental analysis of costs and outcomes
    - sensitivity analyses for uncertainty in costs and outcomes

Box 3.5 Example of tabulation and graphic presentation of study quality assessment

Free form question: Among infertile couples with subfertility due to a male factor, does anti-oestrogen treatment increase pregnancy rates?

Structured question

- The population — Couples with subfertility due to a male factor (low sperm count)
- The interventions — Anti-oestrogen treatment (clomiphene citrate or tamoxifen) for the male partner
  Comparator: placebo, no treatment, or vitamin C
- The outcomes — Pregnancy (critical)
- The study design — Experimental studies

Tabulation of study quality

Information about quality items can be placed in columns with the studies in rows (sorted according to year of publication).

| Author | Year | Randomization | | Blinding | Descripton of withdrawals | Population complete work-up | Outcome 1-year long follow-up | Rank order of quality* |
		Sequence generation	Concealment					
Roonberg	1980	Unstated	Unstated	Unclear	Adequate	Adequate	Inadequate	3
Abel	1982	Unclear	Unclear	Inadequate	Adequate	Unclear	Inadequate	4
Wang	1983	Unclear	Unclear	Inadequate	Unclear	Adequate	Adequate	6
Torok	1985	Unclear	Unclear	Unclear	Unclear	Inadequate	Adequate	5
Micic	1985	Unclear	Unclear	Inadequate	Unclear	Inadequate	Inadequate	9
AinMelk	1987	Unclear	Unclear	Unclear	Unclear	Inadequate	Inadequate	8
Sokol	1988	Adequate	Adquate	Adequate	Unclear	Adequate	Adequate	1
WHO	1992	Adequate	Adequate	Adequate	Adequate	Adequate	Inadequate	2
Karuse	1992	Unclear	Unclear	Inadequate	Unclear	Inadequate	Inadequate	7

* see text for an explanation

Bar chart of study quality

Information on quality presented as 100% stacked bars. Data in the stacks represents the number of studies meeting the quality criteria

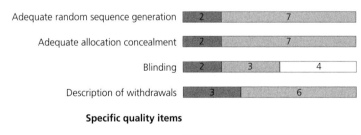

Generic quality items

- Adequate random sequence generation: 2 | 7
- Adequate allocation concealment: 2 | 7
- Blinding: 2 | 3 | 4
- Description of withdrawals: 3 | 6

Specific quality items

- Complete diagnostic work-up: 4 | 1 | 4
- Adequate follow-up duration to detect pregnancies: 3 | 6

0%   25%   50%   75%   100%

Compliance with quality items

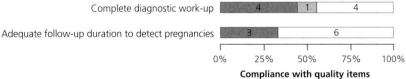

■ Yes ▨ Unclearly reported ☐ No

*Based on Arch Intern Med 1996; **156(6)**: 661–6.*
See Box 4.7 for use of study quality assessment in exploring heterogenity.

in evidence synthesis (Step 4) and interpretation (Step 5). However, reviews including studies with multiple *designs* need not be confusing, particularly if due attention can be given to the quality assessment issues.

When using the approach described in Box 3.1 we might find that in some reviews, where the question demands studies of various designs to be included, the quality assessment will not be so straightforward. A mixture of studies with different designs may become part of a review because more than one design is needed to address the same question or because more than one question is to be addressed. Case study 3 presents an example where studies of both experimental (randomized and non-randomized) and observational (cohort study with concurrent controls) designs are included in a review to address a question about effectiveness. Here it is possible to develop and use a single checklist for quality assessment (Boxes C3.3 and C3.4). Some reviewers prefer to use separate checklists for different designs and this is the most reasonable approach in some situations; for example, when a review addresses two separate but related questions, e.g. about clinical effectiveness and efficiency of an *intervention*. This is like having two reviews in one. Here different quality assessments will have to be developed for the different *study designs* relevant to the two questions, as shown in Box 3.4.

Effectiveness is the extent to which an *intervention* (therapy, prevention, diagnosis, screening, education, social care, etc.) produces beneficial *outcomes* under ordinary day-to-day circumstances.

Efficiency (cost-effectiveness) is the extent to which the balance between input (costs) and outputs (*outcomes*) of *interventions* represents value for money.

3.3 Reliability of the study quality checklist in a review

The evaluation of quality items is very often affected by vague and ambiguous reporting in the selected studies. In order to avoid subjectivity and errors when extracting information about quality, the review protocol should provide a clear description of how to assess quality. This would mean designing data extraction forms with clear and consistent coding of responses. Ideally the forms should be piloted using several reviewers and a sample of studies to assess the reliability of the quality assessment process. Pilot testing might identify confusion about the extraction and coding instructions, which would then need to be clarified – a more explicit system of coding would improve inter-reviewer agreement.

In the past, people have suggested blinding the reviewers to the names of the authors, institutions, journals and year of publication when assessing quality. This should avoid bias as judgements about quality may be unduly influenced by these factors. Therefore some reviewers go to great lengths to have such identifying information masked before examining the manuscripts. However, the cumbersome and time-consuming procedures required to produce blinded papers have not been shown to impact on the conclusions of reviews and unmasked independent quality assessment by more than one reviewer should be sufficient. By now it should be quite clear that it is unwise to undertake a review without co-authors.

3.4 Using study quality assessments in a review

Having developed our checklist and extracted the relevant data on quality assessment, we are ready to integrate this information in our review (Box 3.1). How would we describe the quality of the studies? There are many imaginative ways of presenting information about how the studies included in a review have complied with the quality items. Examples of quality description are shown in the case studies. We may start by describing how many studies meet the various quality criteria and support this with graphs, e.g. using stacked bar charts (Box 3.5). However, tabulation of the information on quality items for each one of the included studies is the clearest way to describe quality (Box 3.5).

One difficult issue in quality assessment is that of ranking studies according to their quality. A simple way is to rank studies according to the proportion of total items they comply with. When studies satisfy the same proportion of quality items, but are deficient in different areas, there is a problem. Here the deficient areas should guide us about the rank: studies with deficiencies in areas with a greater potential for bias (e.g. lack of concealment of allocation) should be ranked lower than those with deficiencies in areas with a smaller risk (e.g. deficiencies in allocation sequence generation). Weighting of items has been proposed but there are no agreed weighting schemes that apply universally. This is because the importance of quality items varies from topic to topic. For example, blinding is highly crucial in studies with subjective *outcomes*, but not so much in those with objective *outcomes*.

Reviewers have to use their judgement when ranking studies according to quality in the context of their topic. For example, in a review concerning effectiveness of a treatment for infertility (Box 3.5), two studies (Sokol and WHO) comply with five out of six quality items. Sokol is 'unclear' about its description of withdrawals and WHO has not followed participants up for one year (in fact they only followed up to 8 months). If we feel that adequacy of follow-up is more important than lack of clarity about the description of withdrawals, then we can rank Sokol higher than WHO. This subjectivity cannot be removed from reviewing, so it is important that judgements are made before the results of the studies are known. This example should also make it clear that there are limits to how detailed judgements can be. Often it is impossible to have a sensible ranking of studies according to quality and one may have to settle for a more crude categorization, e.g. high *versus* low quality studies, as in Case study 2. Having performed quality assessments in a sensible (and unbiased) manner, one can confidently proceed to data synthesis (Step 4), interpretation of results and generation of inferences (Step 5) where variation in the quality of the selected studies may have important implications. We see examples of how strength of evidence is linked to study quality assessment in Box 5.3 and Case studies 7 and 8.

Summary of Step 3: Assessing quality of the literature

Key points about appraising review articles

- Examine the methods section to see if a study quality assessment has been undertaken.
- Has quality been used as a criterion for study selection? (Step 2)
- Has a more detailed assessment of the selected studies been carried out? Are the quality items appropriate for the question? Check the results section and the tables to see how much variation in quality there is between studies.
- Is the variation in quality an explanation for heterogeneity? Is meta-analysis appropriate given the quality? (Step 4)
- Is the strength of the collated evidence linked to quality? (Step 5)

Key points for conducting reviews

- Obsession with quality is the 'Achilles' heel' of all research studies and reviews. Study quality assessment plays a role in every Step of a review.
- Question formulation (Step 1) and study selection criteria (Step 2) should have *study design* components in them to determine the minimum acceptable level of study quality.
- For a more refined quality assessment of selected studies, checklists should be developed which consider the generic issues relevant to the *study design* aspects of the review question. These items may be derived from existing critical appraisal guides and *design*-based quality checklists.
- It is important to consider issues relevant to the *populations*, *interventions* and *outcomes* specific to the question. Considering these specific issues, the existing generic items may be modified or deleted and new relevant items may be added to the quality checklists.
- These detailed quality assessments will be used for describing the selected studies, exploring an explanation for heterogeneity (Step 4), making informed decisions regarding suitability of meta-analysis (Step 4), assessing the strength of the collated evidence (Step 5) and making recommendations for future research.

● Step 4: *Summarizing the evidence*

Step 1
Framing questions
↓
Step 2
Identifying relevant
literature
↓
Step 3
Assessing quality of
the literature
↓
Step 4
Summarizing the
evidence
↓
Step 5
Interpreting the
findings

Collating the findings of studies included in a review requires more than just tabulation and meta-analysis of their results. It requires a deeper exploration and an in-depth analysis, for which the findings need to be presented in a clear way. We need to evaluate whether the observed effects of *interventions* are consistent among the included studies, and if not, why not? We need to assess if a statistical combination of individual effects (meta-analysis) is feasible and appropriate. These analyses allow us to generate meaningful conclusions from the reviews. This Step covers the basics of producing evidence summaries in systematic reviews, limiting the discussion to questions about the effects of *interventions* or *exposures* on binary *outcomes*. Once the principles are understood, they can be applied with appropriate tailoring to other question types (see Case studies 4, 5 and 6).

Effect is a measure of association between an *intervention* or *exposure* and an *outcome*. The term **individual effects** means effects observed in individual studies included in a review. **Summary effect** means the effect generated by pooling individual effects in a meta-analysis.

4.1 Description of data contained in the included studies

To begin with, a descriptive summary of the findings of studies included in a review is required. In simple terms, the objective of this initial exercise is to present (in a meaningful way) the information about studies' characteristics (*populations*, *interventions* and *outcomes*), their *design* and quality, and their effects. There is no need to use any advanced statistics at this stage. We may use tables, figures and simple computations, such as proportions, relative risks, etc, which allow us to glance at the evidence and to glean the differences between studies. This is a crucial part of evidence synthesis; it will help us gain a deeper understanding of the evidence and should prevent errors in interpretation. It will also enhance the transparency of our analysis.

When faced with large amounts of data to be summarized, tabulation can be a daunting task. The process of carrying out the tabulations should follow from the review question. The nature and complexity of the table depends a great deal on how many studies are included and how much data needs to be displayed from each. The decisions about the structure of the tables should be guided by what we considered to be important issues at the time of question formulation and what, in our judgement, could produce a variation in effects (as outlined in Step 1). So, for example, information may be tabulated with studies in rows grouped according to a characteristic of the *population*. Then information on *interventions*, *outcomes* and effects for each study could be summarized succinctly (Box 4.1). Information on

Box 4.1 Tabulating information from studies included in a systematic review

Suggested steps

1. Place features related to populations, interventions and outcomes in columns.
2. Consider what subgroups of populations there are among included studies.
3. Consider what subtypes of interventions there are.
4. Consider the outcomes and their importance.
5. Consider if studies need to be subclassified according to study designs and quality.
6. Populate the cells in the table with information from studies along rows in subgroups.
7. Sort studies according to a feature that helps to understand their results (e.g. a characteristic of a population or intervention, rank order of quality, year of publication, etc).

An example of tabulation of studies in a review of antimicrobials for chronic wounds

This is only a brief tabulation. Detailed tables can be found in the report of the review available at www.hta.nhsweb.nhs.uk/htapubs.htm

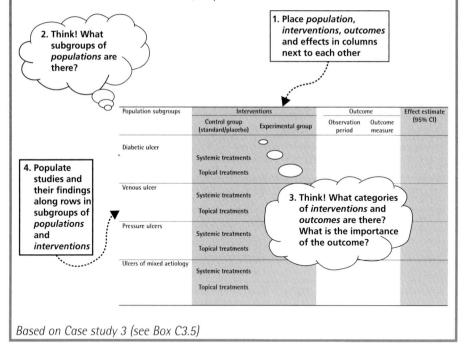

Based on Case study 3 (see Box C3.5)

outcomes should make clear the importance attached to each outcome separately.

Sometimes tables will end up with too many columns to fit on one page. In this situation it is often helpful to breakdown the tabulation into several tables. We may produce one detailed table of *population* characteristics and relevant prognostic factors; another table may include details of *interventions* and yet another for details of *outcomes*. The features of *study designs* and other aspects of study quality may be presented in a separate table or a figure (Box 3.5). Preparation of tables is often laborious and time consuming, but without them we cannot understand the results of the included studies. Once the hard work is done, a quick scan through these tables should allow us, and more importantly others, to judge how studies differ in terms of *populations*, *interventions*, *outcomes* and quality.

At this stage, we should also compute and tabulate the effects found in each one of the studies along with their confidence intervals (Box 4.2). This will help us examine the direction and magnitude of effect among the individual studies. By direction of effect we mean either benefit or harm. By magnitude we mean how much benefit or how much harm. Box 4.3 shows how to evaluate direction and magnitude of effect graphically in a Forest plot.

A simple tabulation of numerical results, like the one shown in Case study 3 (Box C3.5), is not easy to assimilate at a glance. Therefore, it is worth examining effects graphically (Box 4.3). These graphic summaries would help us make qualitative judgements about the effects of *interventions*, particularly about the direction, magnitude and precision of individual effects. Occasionally, this may produce a surprise: a conclusion about effectiveness may be reached solely from qualitative examination of the observed effects without the need for statistical analysis, particularly if there are numerous studies with consistent and large effects. In this situation a quantitative synthesis (meta-analysis) may not add anything to our inferences. However, often the effects will not be precise enough because of a small sample size in individual studies. The graphic display will give us a good idea about effectiveness but this will not be sufficient to generate inferences. Here, meta-analysis will be useful, as it will improve the precision of the effect by statistically combining the results from individual studies – but first we need to assess if the effects vary from study to study (heterogeneity) and if it is sensible to undertake a meta-analysis.

One aim of data description is to assess the extent of the evidence in order to plan statistical analyses. We should have planned our analyses for heterogeneity and meta-analysis in advance, and armed with information from the tables we should be able to assess their feasibility. We will be able to see if data on clinically important *outcomes* are available for the *interventions* we wanted to compare. We may become aware of additional issues of importance, which were not known at the planning stage. If we decide to pursue these issues, we should be honest about reporting them as post-hoc analyses and we should be conscious of the problems of spurious significance associated with them. Our enquiry might be limited due to lack of data or due to missing information on important issues. It might be useful to contact the authors of individual studies before proceeding further; alternatively we could plan a sensitivity analysis to take account of the uncertainties due to missing or unclear information.

Point estimate of effect is its observed value in a study.

Confidence interval is the imprecision in the point estimate, i.e. the range around it within which the 'true' value of the effect can be expected to lie with a given degree of certainty (e.g. 95%).

Point estimate

Confidence interval

The **direction of effect** indicates a beneficial or a harmful effect. The point estimate of effect tells us about direction and magnitude of effect.

The **precision of effect** relates to the degree of uncertainty in the estimation of effect that is due to the play of chance. The confidence interval tells us about precision.

Sensitivity analysis involves repetition of an analysis under different assumptions to examine the impact of these assumptions on the results.

Box 4.2 Estimation of effects observed in individual studies included in a systematic review

Measures of effect

An effect is a statistic, which provides a measure of the strength of relationship between an intervention and an outcome, e.g. relative risk (RR), odds ratio (OR) or risk difference (RD) for binary data; mean difference or standardized mean difference for continuous data; and hazard ratio for survival data (see glossary). Statistical significance tells us nothing about the magnitude of the effect. Effect measures help us to make judgements about the magnitude and clinical importance of the effects. The term individual effects means effects observed in individual studies included in a review. Summary effect means the effect generated by pooling individual effects in a meta-analysis.

Computing effect measures for binary outcomes in individual studies

Computing point estimates of effects is relatively simple, as shown below. With several studies to compute effects for, and to estimate confidence intervals for, every effect makes manual calculation tedious. We would suggest you use a statistical software package. We have generally used RevMan, the Cochrane Collaboration's review management software, to compute and present results in this book (www.cochrane.org/cochrane/revman.htm).

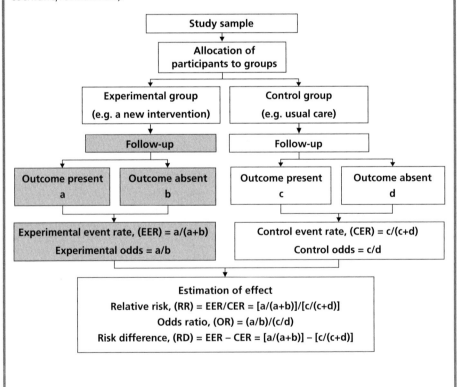

Choosing an effect for binary outcomes

The choice depends on the ease of interpretation and statistical properties of the effect measure. Clinicians prefer relative risk (RR) and number needed to treat (NNT) – which is the inverse of risk difference (RD) – because they are intuitive. Some statisticians prefer OR because it is not sensitive to the reversibility of the event classification and it is more suitable for statistical manipulation and modelling. RR and OR are relative measures of effect and, compared to RD, they tend to be more consistent in systematic reviews when studies have considerable variation in control event rate. The summary NNT (and summary RD) values generated from meta-analyses can be challenging as their meaningful clinical application depends on the knowledge of baseline rates in the *populations* where the results are to be applied (see Step 5). We will often be faced with OR in the medical literature. From these we can generate NNTs for interpretation as shown in Box 5.4.

Box 4.3 Summarizing the effects observed in studies included in a systematic review

Forest plot

This is a commonly used, easy to understand, graphical display of individual effects observed in studies included in a systematic review (along with the summary effect if meta-analysis is used, as in Box 4.4). For each study, a box representing the point estimate of effect lies in the middle of a horizontal line which represents the confidence interval of the effect. When using relative risk (RR) or odds ratio (OR) as the effect measure, the effects are usually plotted on a log-scale. This produces symmetrical confidence intervals around the point estimates. A vertical line drawn at an RR or OR value of 1.0 represents 'no effect'. For desirable outcomes (e.g. pregnancy among infertile couples) RR or OR value > 1.0 indicates that the experimental intervention is effective in improving that outcome compared to the control intervention. However, most reviews report undesirable outcomes (e.g. death) and then RR or OR values < 1.0 indicate an advantage for the experimental group. When using mean difference the value 0 indicates 'no effect'. A confidence interval overlapping the vertical line of 'no effect' represents lack of a statistically significant effect.

Description of effects and their uncertainty in a systematic review

Free form question: Among infertile couples with subfertility due to a male factor, does anti-oestrogen treatment increase pregnancy rates? *(see structured question in Box 3.5)*

The effects observed among nine studies

Effects summarized as RR and OR, sorted by year of publication. Effect values > 1.0 indicate an advantage for the treatment group compared to control, i.e. pregnancy rates improve with anti-oestrogen treatment.

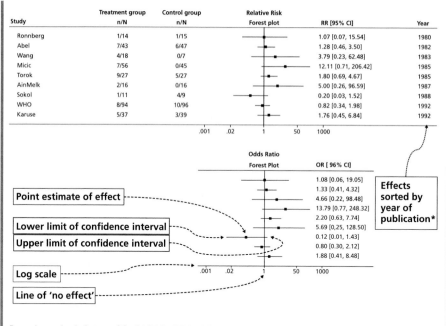

Study	Treatment group n/N	Control group n/N	Relative Risk Forest plot	RR [95% CI]	Year
Ronnberg	1/14	1/15		1.07 [0.07, 15.54]	1980
Abel	7/43	6/47		1.28 [0.46, 3.50]	1982
Wang	4/18	0/7		3.79 [0.23, 62.48]	1983
Micic	7/56	0/45		12.11 [0.71, 206.42]	1985
Torok	9/27	5/27		1.80 [0.69, 4.67]	1985
AinMelk	2/16	0/16		5.00 [0.26, 96.59]	1987
Sokol	1/11	4/9		0.20 [0.03, 1.52]	1988
WHO	8/94	10/96		0.82 [0.34, 1.98]	1992
Karuse	5/37	3/39		1.76 [0.45, 6.84]	1992

.001   .02   1   50   1000

Odds Ratio Forest Plot — OR [96% CI]

Point estimate of effect
Lower limit of confidence interval
Upper limit of confidence interval
Log scale
Line of 'no effect'

1.08 [0.06, 19.05]
1.33 [0.41, 4.32]
4.66 [0.22, 98.48]
13.79 [0.77, 248.32]
2.20 [0.63, 7.74]
5.69 [0,25, 128.50]
0.12 [0.01, 1.43]
0.80 [0.30, 2.12]
1.88 [0.41, 8.48]

Effects sorted by year of publication*

.001   .02   1   50   1000

Based on *Arch Intern Med* 1996; **156**: 661–666

Review manager software used to compute effects and produce graphics (http://www. cochrane.org/cochrane/revman.htm). It is developed by the Cochrane Collaboration and is available as a free download. Technical support is provided only for Cochrane reviewers

*See Box 4.7 for a Forest plot with studies sorted according to rank order of quality

4.2 Investigating differences in effects between studies

There are usually some differences between studies in the key characteristics of their *populations, interventions* and *outcomes* (clinical heterogeneity), and their *study designs* and quality (methodological heterogeneity). These are discovered during tabulation of information from the studies. These variations in study characteristics and quality are likely to have some influence on the observed effects. Investigation of heterogeneity is about this variation of effects between studies and its reasons.

We may begin exploring for the possibility of heterogeneity of effects between studies by studying the tables we produced earlier. However, we will probably get a better idea about heterogeneity by visually examining the Forest plot for variations in effects (Box 4.3). In general, if the point estimates of effects lie on one side of the 'line of no effect', then the *interventions* can be expected to produce the same qualitative effect, either benefit or harm. If the point estimates are located on both sides of the 'line of no effect', then they could produce beneficial and harmful effects (as

Question components
The population: A clinically suitable sample of patients
The interventions: Comparison of groups with and without the intervention
The outcomes: Changes in health status due to interventions
The study design: Ways of conducting research to assess the effect of interventions

in Box 4.3). Clearly this should raise suspicion about heterogeneity. We should also see if the confidence intervals of the effects overlap each other. If they do, as in Box 4.3, then it is more likely that any differences in the point estimates of effects are merely due to chance or indicate only limited heterogeneity, which is unavoidable.

Formal statistical tests for heterogeneity examine if the observed variability in effects is compatible with that expected to occur by chance alone. The chi-square test for heterogeneity among the effects shown in Box 4.3 has a p-value of 0.36 – well above the conventional threshold of $p < 0.05$. These tests tend to have low power so they might miss important between-study differences in effects. It has therefore been suggested that a less stringent threshold of $p < 0.1$ should be used to statistically assess heterogeneity. The formal assessment with the p-value has a serious drawback. The underlying chi-square statistic which leads to the p-value, let's call it Q, has no intuitive meaning. Q increases as the number of included studies, k, increases. To have a more appropriate tool for the assessment of heterogeneity, $I^2 = (Q - (k-1))/Q$ has been introduced. I^2 is interpreted as the proportion of the existing variability due to heterogeneity between studies. I^2 ranges between 0% and 100%; 0% indicates no observed heterogeneity, and larger values show increasing heterogeneity. Values of 25%, 50% and 75% may be taken to represent low, moderate and high levels of heterogeneity. With I^2 dependence on the number of included studies is avoided. However, I^2 still hinges on the precision of the studies, or in other words, on the size of the studies. This limits the use of I^2 when comparing values across meta-analyses with different study sizes.

Assessment of heterogeneity is a challenge in synthesis of studies. There remain many disputes between methodologists about interpretation of heterogeneity statistics and details of these are beyond the scope of this book. A reasonable approach would be to evaluate both informal, non-statistical assessment of heterogeneity (e.g. with the Forest plot) and the I^2 statistic without reliance on p-values alone. Whenever we suspect substantial heterogeneity, we should seek an explanation, whether or not heterogeneity is statistically confirmed. We will turn to exploring reasons for heterogeneity shortly, but first we take a look at the basics of meta-analysis.

Heterogeneity is the variation of effects between studies. It may arise because of differences in key characteristics of their *populations*, *interventions* and *outcomes* (clinical heterogeneity), or their study *designs* and quality (methodological heterogeneity).

Power is the ability of a test to statistically demonstrate a difference when one exists. When a test has low power, a larger sample size is required, otherwise there is a risk that a possible difference might be missed.

I^2 is a statistic ranging from 0% to 100% that gives the percentage of total variation across studies due to heterogeneity.

4.3 Meta-analysis (quantitative synthesis) of effects observed in studies

As indicated earlier, individual studies may be far too small to produce precise effects and so meta-analysis can improve precision by combining them statistically. First we must determine

Meta-analysis is a statistical technique for combining the individual effects of a number of studies addressing the same question to produce a summary effect.

if meta-analysis is at all possible, and if so, whether it would be appropriate. By examining the tables produced for describing the studies we will be able to determine if the data necessary to perform a meta-analysis are available. Sometimes meta-analysis will just not be feasible, for example, when there are important differences between the studies in terms of *populations*, *interventions*, *outcomes* and quality, it would be senseless to try to estimate a summary effect (as in Case study 3). A systematic review does not always have to have a meta-analysis! In addition, by examining for differences in effects between studies, we will be able to determine whether or not the studies are too heterogeneous to be sensibly combined. We should proceed with meta-analysis only if the studies are similar in clinical characteristics and methodological quality, and are homogeneous in effects.

In a meta-analysis, in simple terms, the effects observed across studies are pooled to produce a weighted average effect of all the studies – the summary effect. As a general principal, each study is weighted according to some measure of its importance, e.g. a method that gives more weight to more informative studies (often larger studies with precise effect estimates) and less weight to less informative studies (often smaller studies with imprecise effect estimates) is used. In most meta-analyses, this is achieved by assigning a weight to each study in inverse proportion to the variance, expressing precision, of its effect. Averaging effects across studies in this way ensures that the *intervention* groups within each study are only compared to the control groups in the same study. Thus, in a meta-analysis of experimental studies, the benefit accrued by randomization (with allocation concealment) is preserved when the results are pooled. An example meta-analysis is shown in Box 4.4.

It is important to be familiar with the finer points concerning pooling individual effects in a meta-analysis because we will be faced with them regularly when reading or conducting reviews. During a meta-analysis it is essential to check how robust our summary effect is to the variation in statistical methods. There are two concepts to keep in mind: the 'fixed effect' and 'random effects' statistical models.

A fixed effect model estimates the average effect assuming that there is a single 'true' underlying effect. A random effects model assumes that there is no single underlying value of the effect, but there is a distribution of effects depending on the studies' characteristics. The differences between effects are considered to arise from between-study variation and the play of chance (random variability). A random effects model weights smaller studies proportionally higher than a fixed effect model when estimating a summary effect. This phenomenon may exaggerate the impact of publication bias and poor quality in smaller studies.

When computing confidence intervals, random effects models

Variance is statistical measure of variation measured in terms of deviations of the individual observations from the mean value.

The **inverse of variance** of observed individual effects is often used to weight studies in statistical analyses used in systematic reviews, e.g. meta-analysis, meta-regression and funnel plot analysis.

Box 4.4 Summarizing the effects using meta-analysis

Forest plot of individual and summary effects

Effects observed in individual studies are plotted along with the summary effect. For each study, the point estimate of effect is a box of variable size according to the weight of the study in the meta-analysis. The summary effect is plotted below the individual effects using a different graphic pattern, e.g. a filled diamond (the width of the diamond represents the confidence interval and the centre of the diamond represents the point estimate).

An example meta-analysis using fixed and random effects models

The example shown below is based on the question and the effects (relative risk, RR) described in Box 4.3. Compared to the fixed effect models, the random effects models produce wider confidence interval around the summary effect because they take into account between-study variability. They also preferentially weight smaller studies, which have more varied effects than larger studies.

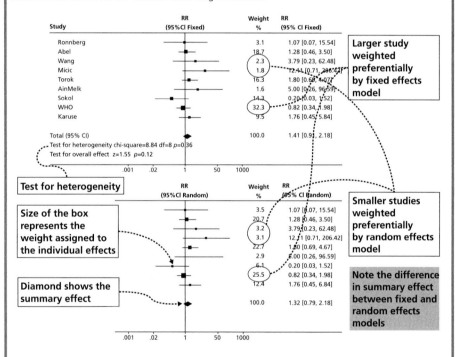

Based on *Arch Intern Med* 1996; **156**: 661–6

Review manager software used to compute effects and produce graphics
See Box 4.7 for subgroup meta-analysis

incorporate the variance of effects observed between the studies (assuming that they have a normal distribution). Hence, when there is heterogeneity, a random effects model produces wider confidence intervals of the summary effect compared with a fixed effect model. Therefore it can be argued that the fixed effect model may give undue precision to the summary effect (spuriously narrow confidence interval) if there is significant unexplained heterogeneity between the studies. In the example meta-analysis shown in Box 4.4 summary effects generated with both fixed and random effects models are demonstrated. In practice both statistical models may be used to assess the robustness of the statistical synthesis, but if we have to make a choice we should do this *a priori* and not after we have been biased by knowledge of the results.

4.4 Clinical heterogeneity

Differences in the characteristics of the studies with respect to *populations*, *interventions* and *outcomes* can provide useful answers regarding heterogeneity and can help in interpreting the clinical relevance of the findings. The exploration of these differences can be facilitated by constructing the summary tables in such a way that potential explanations for differences in effects can be more easily identified. During question formulation (Step 1), we would have identified important issues that could produce a variation in effects (see examples in Box 1.3). Based on this information, we may stratify the studies into subgroups according to *populations*, *interventions* and *outcomes* sets. The differences in effects in the various subgroups of studies can then be explored.

   If there are many studies in our review, the differences in effects may also be examined statistically, as shown in Box 4.5. We can perform a meta-analysis of subgroups of studies and additionally examine if the effects are consistent within the subgroups. Advanced statisticians could also determine the statistical significance (*p*-value) of the difference in the effect between subgroups; this is beyond the scope of this book. We should be aware that investigations into the reasons for heterogeneity must be interpreted with caution. As with statistical tests for detection of heterogeneity, tests for evaluating its reasons also have limited power so they may miss a relationship. Another problem is that if subgroup analyses are carried out, some might be spuriously significant, a problem inherent in multiple analyses of any type.

Box 4.5 Exploring clinical heterogeneity

Subgroup analysis

Free form question: Do home visits improve the health of elderly people?

Structured question

● The populations	Elderly people in various age groups
● The interventions	Home visits of various intensities and frequencies
	Comparator: usual care
● The outcomes	Mortality, functional status and nursing home admissions
● The study design	Experimental studies

Delineation of various subgroups (*considering the detailed question structure in Box 1.3*)

Subgroups	1 Age-based subgroups	2 Assessment intensity based subgroups	3 Follow-up frequency based subgroups
● The populations	Elderly people in various age groups	Elderly people	Elderly people
● The interventions	Home visits	Home visits of various assessment intensities	Home visits of various frequencies of follow-up
	Comparator: usual care.	Comparator: usual care.	Comparator: usual care.
● The outcomes	Mortality (critical)	Functional status (critical)	Nursing home admissions (important)

Subgroup meta-analyses

A vertical line in the centre of the diamond indicates the point estimate of the summary relative risk (RR) for each subgroup of studies with particular characteristics. The width of the diamond represents the confidence interval of the summary RR for each subgroup. RR values of < 1.0 represent an advantage for the intervention group compared to control.

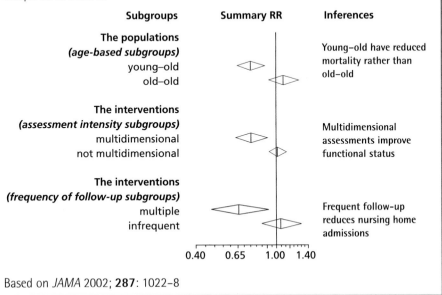

Based on *JAMA* 2002; **287**: 1022–8

Therefore examination of the explanation for heterogeneity should be planned for a small number of study characteristics for which there is a strong suggestion of a relationship with the size of effect.

In addition, the choice of subgroups should be made in advance (Step 1). It is good to be cautious – from examining the tables we generated earlier we might become aware of issues and possible relationships we had not anticipated. The temptation would be to undertake further subgroup analyses that were not originally planned. These post-hoc analyses should be avoided. If we cannot resist the temptation, they should be clearly identified and their findings should be interpreted cautiously. They should not be used to guide clinical practice but they can be used to generate hypotheses for testing in future research.

Where substantial heterogeneity is present and clinical reasons for it can be found, an overall meta-analysis may be unnecessary. In this situation, meta-analysis should be restricted to clinically relevant subgroups where a variation in effect was originally anticipated. This approach will aid in clinical interpretation and application of the review's findings as highlighted by the example shown in Box 4.5.

4.5 Methodological heterogeneity

We should also find out if *design* and quality differences among studies appear to be associated with variation in their effects. This is important not only to explore reasons for heterogeneity, but also to assess the strength of the evidence (Step 5).

Hopefully, *study design* will have been used as one of the selection criteria (Step 2). This way studies of poor *design* would have been removed and the review would have focused on studies of a minimum acceptable quality from the outset. So why should there be a fuss about the quality of a review's component studies? In many reviews, depending on the type and amount of available literature, it is inevitable that selection criteria specifying the *study design* will allow inclusion of studies of methodologically inferior *designs* (Step 2). Even when search and selection focus on robust *study designs*, there will be some variation in quality between studies. This happens because the devil about quality is in the detail: the 'gross' hierarchies of *study designs* used for study selection do not capture finer points about quality which are important for the validity of the results.

Hopefully, we would have performed detailed study quality assessments and discovered the variation in quality between studies (Step 3). During study synthesis we should gauge if quality has an association with the estimation of effects as part of the exploration for heterogeneity and its sources. The reason for being concerned about study quality is that if we find different individual effects among studies of different quality, we can no longer trust the overall summary effect. If high quality studies produce conservative estimates of effect, our inferences would also have to be conservative.

We may have got some idea about the relationship between

> The **quality** of a study depends on the degree to which its design, conduct and analysis minimizes **biases**.

> **Bias** either exaggerates or underestimates the 'true' effect of an *intervention* or *exposure*.

quality and effects by tabulating the relevant information on quality and effects together. In fact, where studies of different *designs* are included in a review, we should tabulate the studies subgrouped according to *design*. In this situation, if a meta-analysis is (mistakenly) undertaken using studies of different *designs*, there is a risk that biased summary effects may be produced due to undue weighting of studies that are inferior in *design*. In an attempt to counter such a bias, the idea of weighting studies in proportion to their quality (rather than size or precision as described earlier) has been suggested. However, no agreed standards exist for producing such weights, so we should abandon this idea. Sometimes the only feasible approach will be a descriptive evidence summary, particularly if there are no subgroups of studies of a similar quality, but if there are, use a subgroup meta-analysis.

A meta-analysis should only be contemplated within subgroups of studies of the same *design* and inferences should be based on the effects observed among studies of superior *design*. As shown in Box 4.6, we might find that studies of superior *designs* do not show an association between *exposure* and *outcome* when studies of inferior *designs* do. Even when a review focuses on studies of a single *design*, there may be variation in effects according to quality. Often the relationship between quality and effect would result in heterogeneity, but this is by no means the rule. If the studies' effects were stacked in decreasing order of quality in a Forest plot, the relationship would become apparent. For example, an increase in effect may be observed as the quality deteriorates, as shown in Box 4.7.

Box 4.6 Using study design to gauge strength of inferences

Free form question: Is exposure to benzodiazepines during pregnancy associated with malformations in the newborn baby? (*also see Box 1.2*)

Structured question

● The population	Pregnant women
● The exposures	Benzodiazepines in early pregnancy
	Comparator: no exposure
● The outcomes	Major malformations in the newborn baby
● The study design	Observational studies with cohort and case-control designs (*see Box 1.4*)

Summary of evidence

There was statistically significant heterogeneity in the overall analysis. Overall summary odds ratio (OR) suggested a trend towards an association between exposure to benzodiazepines and the risk of major malformations in the newborn baby. We use OR in this analysis because among studies with case-control *design* it is not possible to compute risk and relative risk.

Exploring the impact of study design on the effects observed in the review

Subgroup analysis stratified according to study design

The association between exposure to benzodiazepines in pregnancy and major malformations is only supported by the subgroup of case-control studies (where there is heterogeneity). These studies are of a more inferior design than cohort studies. Among the sub-group of studies with cohort design (where there is no heterogeneity) there is no association.

Note: OR values >1.0 indicate an association of malformations with exposure to benzodiazepines compared to no exposure.

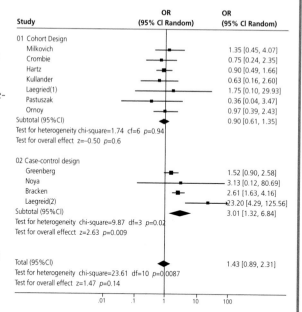

Study	OR (95% CI Random)
01 Cohort Design	
Milkovich	1.35 [0.45, 4.07]
Crombie	0.75 [0.24, 2.35]
Hartz	0.90 [0.49, 1.66]
Kullander	0.63 [0.16, 2.60]
Laegried(1)	1.75 [0.10, 29.93]
Pastuszak	0.36 [0.04, 3.47]
Ornoy	0.97 [0.39, 2.43]
Subtotal (95%CI)	0.90 [0.61, 1.35]

Test for heterogeneity chi-square=1.74 cf=6 p=0.94
Test for overall effect z=−0.50 p=0.6

Study	OR (95% CI Random)
02 Case-control design	
Greenberg	1.52 [0.90, 2.58]
Noya	3.13 [0.12, 80.69]
Bracken	2.61 [1.63, 4.16]
Laegreid(2)	23.20 [4.29, 125.56]
Subtotal (95%CI)	3.01 [1.32, 6.84]

Test for heterogeneity chi-square=9.87 df=3 p=0.02
Test for overall effecct z=2.63 p=0.009

Total (95%CI)	1.43 [0.89, 2.31]

Test for heterogeneity chi-square=23.61 df=10 p=0.0087
Test for overall effect z=1.47 p=0.14

Naïve inference without considering study design

Exposure to benzodiazepines in pregnancy is possibly associated with major malformations in the newborn baby.

Inference considering study design

Exposure to benzodiazepines in pregnancy is *not* associated with major malformations in the newborn baby.

Based on Dolovich *et al. BMJ* 1998; **317**: 839–43

RevMan software used to compute effects and produce graphics
See Box 4.4 for summarizing effects using meta-analysis

Box 4.7 Using study quality to gauge strength of inferences

Free form question: Among infertile couples with subfertility due to a male factor, does anti-oestrogen treatment increase pregnancy rates? (*see structured question in Box 3.5*)

Summary of evidence (based on the review summaries in Box 4.3 and 4.4)

There was no statistically significant heterogeneity in the overall analysis. Summary relative risk (RR) suggested a trend towards an increase in pregnancy rate among couples treated with anti-oestrogens.

Exploring the impact of study quality on the effects observed in the review

Forest plot with effects stacked in decreasing order of quality*

For high-quality studies there is a trend towards harm from treatment. As the quality of studies decreases this trend reverses and the possibility of benefit emerges.

Subgroup analysis stratified according to quality*

The beneficial trend in the overall meta-analysis is supported only by low-quality studies. High-quality studies suggest a trend towards harm, i.e. decrease in pregnancy rates, with treatment.

Note: RR values >1.0 indicate an advantage for anti-oestrogen treatment compared with control.

See Box 3.5 for detailed quality assessment of individual studies and rank order.

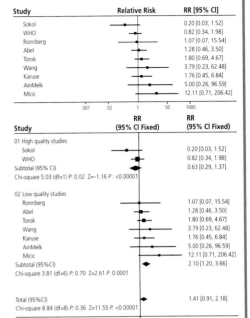

Naïve inference without considering quality
Anti-oestrogen therapy seems to have a trend towards a beneficial effect among infertile couples with subfertility due to a male factor.

Inference considering study quality
Anti-oestrogen therapy has *no* beneficial effect among infertile couples with subfertility due to a male factor.

Based on *Arch Intern Med* 1996; **156(6)**: 661–666

RevMan software used to compute effects and produce graphics
See Box 3.5 for a detailed description of quality
See Box 4.3 for a Forest plot with studies sorted according to year of publication
See Box 4.4 for summarizing effects using meta-analysis

We should explore the relationship between study quality and effects even when heterogeneity is not statistically demonstrable, because effects among high-quality studies may be different from those among low-quality studies (Box 5.3). There is some controversy about how to do this. Some experts consider it preferable to perform a subgroup analysis, stratifying the studies according to their compliance with individual quality items; but this has the disadvantage of increasing the number of subgroups (see Case study 4), which in turn carries the risk of spurious statistical significance. Alternatively, quality scores (composed with the quality items) may be used to stratify studies, but the scoring systems are usually not well developed (Step 3). If there is a good correlation between studies with regard to compliance (and non-compliance) with a number of quality items, it may be sensible to stratify studies into high- and low-quality subgroups based on compliance with most of the quality items (Box 4.7). This approach would reduce the number of subgroup analyses and minimize the risk of spurious findings.

A technique for exploring heterogeneity (called meta-regression) is becoming fashionable, so we should touch on it briefly, mainly with a view to helping us with critical appraisal. Put simply, this technique fits a multivariable linear regression model for examining the influence of study characteristics and quality on the size of individual effects observed among studies included in a review. In this way it searches for the unique contribution of different variables towards an explanation for heterogeneity. Meta-regression does have a down side – it suffers from the risk of what is described in regression analysis as 'overfitting'. This arises because reviews often only have a small number of studies and a large number of variables are available for inclusion in the model. In this situation, if a regression model is used, it will lead to spurious findings. So beware! The most powerful way to assess between-study differences is based on an analysis using individual patient data from the included studies. However, this is only rarely possible.

4.6 Meta-analysis when heterogeneity remains unexplained

Hopefully studies included in our review will not have any obvious heterogeneity. If we do encounter it, hopefully our exploration for reasons behind the heterogeneity will bear some fruit. However, in many reviews there will be no explanations, neither clinical nor methodological. In this situation one might say that heterogeneity remains unexplained despite a sensible exploration. This may be because the number of studies in a review is not large enough to allow a powerful analysis to decipher the reasons behind differences in effects between studies. Now, do we or do we not perform meta-analysis? There is no simple answer.

We should ask ourselves what is to be gained by meta-analysis. Can we not interpret the studies' findings with tabulation and Forest plots of individual effects? The temptation would be to attribute the heterogeneity to chance variation between studies and then undertake meta-analysis using a random effects model as this approach accounts for the variation between studies that cannot be explained by other factors. If we do succumb to this temptation (which happens far too often), proceed with caution. Make sure to look for and exclude funnel asymmetry (Box 4.8), a factor indicative of publication and related biases. Otherwise

Publication bias is said to arise when the likelihood of publication of studies and thus their accessibility to reviewers is related to the significance of their results regardless of their quality.

a random effects model may produce biased summary effect estimates. In addition, our interpretation of the summary effect should be cautious as heterogeneity limits the strength of the evidence collated in reviews (Step 5). We must examine to see if the overall summary effect and the effects of the high-quality subgroup of studies are, by and large, consistent. Even when there is no apparent reason for heterogeneity, the results of high-quality studies may be different. In this way quality becomes a factor in the assessment of strength of evidence (Step 5).

4.7 Exploring for publication and related biases

How can we be sure that our review does not suffer from publication and related biases? Hopefully a systematic approach has been used to track down studies, whether they are published or not (Step 2). Hopefully, the search has particularly focused on capturing those studies that are less accessible, e.g. through searching multiple databases, and has not used language restrictions in study identification. Hopefully, the cast net is wide enough to capture all relevant studies (or at least an unbiased sample of the relevant literature). However thorough the literature search is, there cannot be any guarantees. But there can be some comfort (or discomfort) from formal post-hoc assessment for publication and related biases in a review.

A simple, in many cases too simple, but commonly used method of exploring for these biases is based on the so-called 'funnel plot' analysis. To perform this analysis meaningfully numerous studies, including some large studies, are required. As shown in Box 4.8, it is a scatter plot of individual effects that are observed among studies included in a review against some measure of study information (e.g. study size, inverse of variance). If all the relevant studies ever carried out are included in our review, the scatter of data points in the plot can be expected to lie within a symmetric funnel shape. The funnel is inverted when the y-axis is taken to represent study size (or inverse of variance), as in Box 4.8. This is because there is a wider range of effects among smaller studies compared to the effects observed among larger studies, due to less precision in smaller studies. In this situation the funnel therefore is symmetrical and we can have more confidence that publication and related biases are unlikely in our review. If the funnel is truncated (sometimes called banana-shaped), a group of studies may be missing from our review. Usually missing studies are small in size with different effects to those observed in the large studies included in our review. Such omissions are unlikely to be due to chance alone and they make the funnel asymmetrical. Publication bias is just one of a host of related reasons for funnel asymmetry, including location bias, English language bias, database bias, citation bias, multiple publication bias, poor methodological

Variance is a statistical measure of variation, measured in terms of deviation of the individual observations from the mean value.

The **inverse of variance** of observed individual effects is often used to weight studies in the statistical analyses used in systematic reviews, e.g. meta-analysis, meta-regression and funnel plot analysis.

Box 4.8 Funnel plots to explore for publication and related biases

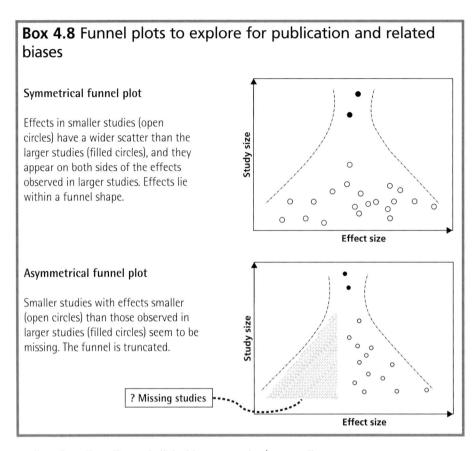

Symmetrical funnel plot

Effects in smaller studies (open circles) have a wider scatter than the larger studies (filled circles), and they appear on both sides of the effects observed in larger studies. Effects lie within a funnel shape.

Asymmetrical funnel plot

Smaller studies with effects smaller (open circles) than those observed in larger studies (filled circles) seem to be missing. The funnel is truncated.

quality of small studies and clinical heterogeneity (e.g. small studies in high risk populations) to name a few. The multiplicity of reasons, and the difficulty in separating them from each other, has led to use of the term small-study-effect rather than publication bias. Whatever the reason, our confidence in the findings of the review will be limited if there is a truncation of the funnel.

A number of statistical tests are available to examine if funnel asymmetry is likely to be due to chance. These are outside the remit of this book, but some advice will be helpful for critical appraisal of reviews. The shapes of funnel plots vary according to the measures of effect and study size, and statistical tests for asymmetry often don't give consistent results. So, to avoid overinterpretation, funnel plot analyses should only be considered exploratory in nature. If it is any consolation, the true extent of publication and related biases may never be known.

Summary of Step 4: Summarizing the evidence

Key points about appraising review articles
- Examine the methods and results sections to see if heterogeneity of effects is evaluated.

- Was the exploration for heterogeneity planned in advance?
- Is variation in clinical characteristics of the studies an explanation for heterogeneity?
- Is variation in study design and quality an explanation for heterogeneity?
- Is meta-analysis appropriate in the light of information gathered on heterogeneity and its reasons?
- Is there a risk of publication and related biases?

Key points about conducting reviews
- The aim of this Step is to collate and summarize the findings of studies included in a review.
- Data synthesis consists of tabulation of study characteristics, quality and effects as well as use of statistical methods for exploring differences between studies and combining their effects (meta-analysis) appropriately.
- Tabulation of evidence helps in assessing feasibility of planned statistical syntheses and improves overall transparency.
- Exploration of heterogeneity and its sources should be planned in advance.
- Exploration of clinical heterogeneity should be based on a small number of study characteristics for which there is a strong theoretical basis for a relationship with estimation of effect.
- Exploration of methodological heterogeneity should consider factors for which there is strong theoretical or empirical basis for suspecting a relationship with bias.
- The following questions should be considered prior to embarking on meta-analysis: Is meta-analysis feasible given clinical heterogeneity? Is meta-analysis feasible given the variation in study quality?
- If an overall quantitative summary is not feasible, subgroup meta-analysis might be feasible and could provide clinically useful answers.
- If feasible, funnel plot analysis should be undertaken to explore for the risk of publication and related biases.

Step 5: Interpreting the findings

Deciphering the salience of a review's findings is as much art as it is science. The ultimate purpose of a review is to inform decision making, and the big question at the end of a systematic review is 'how can one go about making decisions with the collated evidence?' However, the task of generating meaningful and practical answers from reviews is not always easy. We will cover some of the key issues that aid sensible and judicious interpretation of the evidence, avoiding both over- as well as under-interpretation.

Step 1
Framing questions
↓
Step 2
Identifying relevant literature
↓
Step 3
Assessing quality of the literature
↓
Step 4
Summarizing the evidence
↓
Step 5
Interpreting the findings

The Grading of Recommendations Assessment, Development and Evaluation (**GRADE**) working group is an informal collaboration that aims to develop a comprehensive methodology for assessing the strength of the evidence collated in systematic reviews and for generating recommendations from evidence in guidelines. See www.gradeworkinggroup.org. This chapter and interpretation of findings in case studies draws on this methodology.

By the time our review is nearing completion or after having read someone else's review, we may think that we already know the meaning of the findings. But what are the main findings? Is the evidence strong? How much trust can we have in the results of the review? How can we generate inferences and recommendations for current clinical practice as well as for future research? The answers to these questions may not be as straightforward as one might think in the first instance.

This step describes transparent and replicable ways to determine the strength of the evidence collated in a review for generating clinically meaningful and trustworthy bottom lines that aid in application of research into practice.

5.1 Strength of the evidence

How do we gauge the strength of the evidence? This will depend on the strengths and weaknesses of the review. How well did it comply with the key points on appraising reviews at the end of each Step in this book:

Question components
The population: A suitable sample of participants
The exposures: Comparison of groups with and without the exposure
The outcomes: Changes in health status due to interventions
The study design: Ways of conducting research to assess the effect of interventions
The effect: A measure of association between interventions and outcomes

- Is there evidence on critical and important *outcomes* for the *population* and *intervention* of interest described in the question?
- Are the searches adequate?
- Is there a risk of publication and related biases?
- Is the methodological quality of the included studies good enough?
- Are the results consistent from study to study?
- Are there enough data for precise estimation of effect?
- Are the observed effects of substantial clinical, not just statistical, significance?

We have formulated a focused and structured question. We have to compare how well the evidence matches against the components of the question. Were the study *populations* sicker, older or from a different setting? Are *interventions* replicable in our workplace? Have we thought about *outcomes* relevant to patients and classified them as critical, important and less important? (Step 1). Are results available for critical and important *outcomes*? The principal findings should relate to these. Other findings should be considered secondary.

Having undertaken a thorough literature search (Step 2), we have examined the results for publication bias and other related biases (Box 4.8). We have considered the design and quality of studies included in the review (Step 3; Box 3.5). We have explored the observed effects of the individual studies for (in)consistency (Step 4). We have probed whether certain *population* features such as severity of the disease or the setting (Box 4.5), *intervention* features such as treatment intensity or timing (Box 4.5) or methodological features such as study design or study quality (Boxes 4.6 and 4.7) are associated with a larger or reduced size of relative effect. We have inspected the confidence intervals around the effect estimates to evaluate (im)precision.

Having explored in-depth the above issues individually, we ultimately need to make a judgement about the overall strength of the evidence. This judgement should be arrived at in an explicit manner. It would be wise to stop for a moment and consider what we mean by the term 'strength of evidence': In the context of systematic reviews, the strength of the evidence describes the extent to which we can be confident that the estimate of an observed effect is correct for critical and important *outcomes*. The judgements on the strength of the evidence can be classified as being of high, moderate, low or very low level (Box 5.1).

Publication bias is said to arise when the likelihood of a study being published, and thus its accessibility to reviewers, is related to the significance of its results regardless of their quality.

The **direction of effect** indicates a beneficial or a harmful effect. The point estimate of effect tells us about direction and magnitude of effect.

The **precision of effect** relates to the degree of uncertainty in the estimation of effect that is due to the play of chance. The confidence interval tells us about precision.

The **point estimate** of effect is its observed value in a study.

The **confidence interval** is the imprecision in the point estimate, i.e. the range around it within which the 'true' value of the effect can be expected to lie with a given degree of certainty (e.g. 95%).

Point estimate

Confidence interval

Box 5.1 Levels of strength of evidence collated in a review

The strength of evidence describes the extent to which we can be confident that the estimate of an observed effect, i.e. the measure of association between interventions and outcomes assessed in the review, is correct for critical and important questions.

High strength of evidence: We are very confident that the true effect lies close to the observed effect.

Moderate strength of evidence: We are moderately confident that the true effect is likely to be close to the observed effect, but there is a possibility that it could be substantially different.

Low strength of evidence: Our confidence in the observed effect is limited. The true effect may be substantially different from the observed effect.

Very low strength of evidence: We have very little confidence in the observed effect. The true effect is likely to be substantially different from the observed effect.

5.1.1 Assigning a level of strength to evidence

We begin the process of assigning a level of strength to evidence by evaluating the study design (Box 1.4). As a default rule, evidence from experimental design is initially assigned a high level of strength while that from observational design is assigned a low level. Appraisal of key issues concerning directness of evidence in relation to question, publication bias, methodological quality of included studies, and heterogeneity and precision of results is then employed to lower the initially assigned level of strength by one or two levels. This depends, as shown in the examples below, on how much the critical appraisal of key issues alters the confidence in the observed effect.

One has to explicitly consider how good the methodological quality of included studies has to be for evidence to be valid? How consistent should the effects be across studies to be homogeneous? How large should an improvement in effect be for it to be relevant for clinical practice? When is a confidence interval narrow enough to be called precise? Addressing these questions involves judgement, which requires a mixture of methodological and clinical expertise. Whatever the judgement, it should be explicit and transparent, so that others can make sense of the reasoning employed to assign levels of strength of evidence.

Consider Case study 3 for instance, where the included studies are of experimental design. To begin with one may consider the strength of evidence to be at a high level. If the review on antimicrobial therapy in chronic wounds only reported the *outcome* reduction in histologically documented inflammation,

Strength of evidence describes the extent to which we can be confident that the estimate of an observed effect is correct for important questions. It takes into account directness of outcome measure, study design, study quality, heterogeneity, imprecision and publication bias (this is not an exhaustive list).

Heterogeneity is the variation of effects between studies. It may arise because of differences in key characteristics of their *populations*, *interventions* and *outcomes* (clinical heterogeneity), or their study *designs* and quality (methodological heterogeneity).

most would agree there would be difficulties in translating results based on this surrogate into practice. This is because one would prefer to base practice on results from data on a clinically relevant *outcome* like complete wound healing. On reflection, rating down the strength of this evidence by a couple of levels to low because of indirectness of the *outcome* would seem appropriate.

Are there situations where strength of evidence can be justifiably raised after initially assigning a low level? Consider a systematic review of observational studies on the protective effect of bicycle helmets, compared to not wearing such helmets (*Cochrane Database Syst Rev* 1999; Issue 4: CD001855). This demonstrated a strong protective effect against head injury, a critical *outcome*. The effect size measured by OR was 0.31 with a 95% confidence interval of 0.26–0.37. At the outset the level of strength of evidence is considered low due to the risk of bias in observational study design. The bias may inflate the protective effect of the helmet observed in the review. However, it is unlikely that the large observed effect is solely due to the bias inherent in the observational design. The true effect may smaller, but it is unlikely that there would be no protective effect in reality. This raised our confidence in the observed effect and we have good reason for rating up the level of strength of evidence from low to moderate.

Odds ratio (OR) is an effect measure for binary data. It is the ratio of odds in the experimental group to the odds in the control group.

Take, as another example, antibiotic treatment in otitis media (Box 5.2). The review found a reasonably large point estimate of effect. The OR was 0.51 for the critical *outcome* perforation of the ear drum, indicating that the odds of perforation under antibiotics were reduced by half. However, the confidence interval around this point estimate ranged from 0.2 to 1.26, including the possibility of a benefit as large as a reduction in odds by 80%. However, at the other extreme the confidence interval crossed the line of no effect (OR = 1.0) and included the possibility of a 26% increase in the odds of perforation under antibiotics. This result leaves considerable uncertainty about the true effect of antibiotics on perforation. We may, justifiably, make a judgment that this imprecision in the result merits lowering the level of strength of the evidence by a couple of levels, from high to low.

A dose–response relationship would demonstrate that at higher doses the strength of association is increased. This can raise the level of strength of evidence from observational studies. Consider observational studies that consistently show that in patients on oral anticoagulation the risk of bleeding increases with higher INR values. It is needless to say that criteria for raising and relegating the strength level of the evidence should be applied judiciously and transparently.

A **dose–response relationship** demonstrates that at higher doses the strength of association between exposure and outcome is increased.

5.2 Tabulating findings to aid interpretation

To improve transparency, a summary of findings table should be prepared. The results and levels of strength of evidence should be stratified according to the *outcomes*. The number of studies and participants should be included per outcome to illustrate how much the body of evidence varies. The impact of antibiotic therapy in otitis media is investigated by nine studies with 2287 patients for the outcome pain on days 2–7, while only two studies with 381 patients assessed prevention of perforation of the ear drum (Box 5.2).

The strength of the evidence should be evaluated separately for each *outcome*. This is because the strength of the evidence may vary across *outcomes*, even when the evidence comes from the same studies. For example, in the otitis media example (Box 5.3), take the outcome pain at 2–7 days. The strength of the evidence is high because the *populations*, *interventions* and *outcomes* refer directly to the question posed and there are no limitations in the methodological quality of the studies. The results are consistent across studies, the confidence interval around the point estimate of effect is narrow and there is no indication of publication bias. Contrast this with the *outcome* perforation of the ear drum. There is a limitation in study quality, because one large trial excluded from the analysis all patients who had dropped out before this outcome could be addressed. There is imprecision around the observed effect. We have a low level of confidence in the impact of antibiotic therapy on the prevention of perforation.

5.3 Applicability of findings

By this time we must be thinking that we have reached the end. We already know if we can have sufficient trust in the review and we also have a good idea of the magnitude and range of the expected benefits (or harms or other outcomes). However, we need to do a bit more work before applicability of findings can be assessed.

We have measured the effects in relative terms (e.g. relative risk [RR] and odds ratio [OR]) as suggested in Box 4.2. Although the relative effect measures are useful for assessing the strength of the effect (and to perform meta-analysis), to judge whether an intervention is worthwhile, the absolute magnitude of the benefits, tailored to specific population groups, is needed. This allows the clinical significance and the possible impact of the intervention to be understood. The absolute effect might be expressed as the risk difference (RD), which is a fraction, not a whole number (it is sometimes also called 'absolute risk reduction'). The average human brain can only interpret natural frequencies or whole numbers well. The reciprocal of RD converts a fraction into a

Risk difference (RD) is an effect measure for binary data. In a comparative study, it is the difference in event rates between two groups.

Number needed to treat (NNT) is the inverse of RD in individual studies.

Box 5.2 Summary of findings in a review of effectiveness of antibiotics in otitis media among children seen in primary care

Importance of outcome	Outcome	Odds ratio [95% CI]	Baseline risk (risk without treatment)	Risk under treatment* [95% CI]	Risk difference [95% CI]	NNT or NNH+ [95% CI]
Important	**Pain 2–7 days** 9 Trials	0.57 [0.45–0.73]	Medium: 260 per 1000 (26%)	167 per 1000 [137–204]	93 less per 1000 treated [56–123]	11 [8–18]
Critical	**Perforation** (assessed with otoscopy or examination of discharging ear within 7 days follow-up) 2 Trials	0.51 [0.2–1.26]	Low: 17 per 1000 (1.7%)	9 per 1000 [3–21]	8 less per 1000 treated [14 fewer – 4 more]	125 [NNT: 250 – NNH: 71]
			Medium: 160 per 1000 (16%)	89 per 1000 [37–194]	71 less per 1000 treated [123 fewer – 34 more]	14 [NNT: 29 – NNH: 8]
Important	**Adverse effects** (Vomiting, diarrhoea, rash) 4 Trials	1.94 [1.28–2.94]	Low: 10 per 1000 (1%)	19 per 1000 [13–29]	9 more per 1000 treated [3–19]	111 [52–333]
			High: 300 per 1000 (30%)	454 per 1000 [354–558]	154 more per 1000 treated [54–258]	6 [3–18]

* Risk under treatment is based on the risk without treatment and the odds ratio of the intervention calculated using GRADEpro software freely available at www.gradeworkinggroup.org

+ NNT is number needed to treat; NNH is number needed to harm; see Box 5.4 for NNT computation

Box 5.3 Assessing strength of the evidence collated in a review of effectiveness of antibiotics in otitis media among children seen in primary care.

Outcome and its importance	Study design	Directness of outcome measure	Study quality (risk of bias)	Inconsistency of results (heterogeneity)	Imprecision of effects	Publication bias	Strength of evidence
Pain 2–7 days (Important)	Randomized trial *Initially assigned a high strength level*	Direct → No change	No limitations → No change	Consistent → No change	Precise → No change	Not detected → No change	*High*
Perforation (Critical)	Randomized trial *Initially assigned a high strength level*	Direct → No change	Serious limitations → Relegation	Consistent → No change	Imprecise → Relegation	Not assessed → No change	*Low*
Adverse effects (Important)	Randomized trial *Initially assigned a high strength level*	Direct → No change	No limitations → No Change	Consistent → No change	Imprecise → Relegation	Not assessed → No change	*Moderate*

whole number called the number needed to treat (NNT). When dealing with an adverse effect the same calculation is called number needed to harm (NNH). However, this simple approach is only useful in dealing with data from individual studies. When using relative summary effect estimates obtained from reviews, the computation of the NNT is a bit more complicated and freely available software helps with calculation. This is explained in Box 5.4, but first we examine some virtues of NNTs.

Decision making in healthcare is influenced by many factors. The size of the effect and its statistical significance in a meta-analysis provide only part of the information required. For example, when we interpret the summary effect, having received information about our patient's risk of an outcome without treatment, we might decide not to use it in low-risk patients as in our judgement the treatment-associated morbidity and costs may not be worth the benefits. Thus, we may only use the treatment for patients at high risk. Relative effect measures tend to be constant across varying baseline risk, so they are not as informative when tailoring treatment decisions. The NNT, however, is sensitive to changing baseline risks and it allows us to individualize the benefit of interventions. The higher the NNT, the greater the number of patients clinicians must treat to achieve a beneficial effect in one. Therefore they would be less inclined to recommend treatment and their patients would be more inclined to avoid treatment. Very often, in patients at higher baseline risk (i.e. worse prognosis), the NNT will be lower than in patients at lower risk (i.e. good prognosis). The lower the NNT, the smaller the number of patients clinicians must treat to achieve a beneficial result in one person; the more inclined a clinician would be to recommend treatment and the more enthusiastic their patients would be to have treatment.

Baseline risk is the risk of *outcome* in a *population* without *intervention*. It is related to severity of the underlying disease and prognostic factors. Baseline risk is important for determining who will benefit most from an *intervention*.

Prognosis is a probable course or outcome of a disease. Prognostic factors are patient or disease characteristics, which influence the course. Good prognosis is associated with a low rate of undesirable outcomes. Poor prognosis is associated with a high rate of undesirable outcomes.

Box 5.4 Individualizing summary effects from reviews to clinical scenarios

Free form question: Does aspirin in early pregnancy prevent later onset of hypertensive disorders?

Structured question

- The population   Women in early pregnancy
- The interventions   Low dose aspirin
                                  Comparator: placebo or no treatment
- The outcomes   Hypertensive disorders of pregnancy
- The study design   Experimental studies (*see Box 1.4*)

Summary of evidence of effectiveness of aspirin (Based on *BMJ* 2001; 322: 329–33)

There were 32 relevant studies. Aspirin prevented hypertensive disorders of pregnancy with a summary relative risk (RR) of 0.85 (95% confidence interval 0.78–0.92). (RR values < 1.0 indicate an advantage for aspirin treatment compared to control.)

Exploring variation in relative effects of aspirin among various risk groups

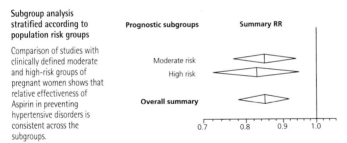

Subgroup analysis stratified according to population risk groups

Comparison of studies with clinically defined moderate and high-risk groups of pregnant women shows that relative effectiveness of Aspirin in preventing hypertensive disorders is consistent across the subgroups.

Individualizing aspirin prevention among various risk groups in early pregnancy

Numbers of women needed to be treated (NNT) with aspirin to prevent hypertension in pregnancy may be computed for various risk groups defined according to the clinical history and the results of the Doppler ultrasound test. This would aid in decision making as one would be quite inclined to treat Doppler-positive women and not so inclined to treat Doppler-negative women according to the following NNTs.

Risk group	Baseline risk*	NNT+
Clinical history: high risk		
Doppler-positive	23.5%	29
Doppler-negative	7.8%	86
Clinical history: moderate risk		
Doppler-positive	18.8%	36
Doppler-negative	2.5%	267

* *Based on a review of diagnostic accuracy of Doppler test in predicting pregnancy hypertension (BJOG 2000; **107**: 196–208)*

+ *Computed using the following formula:*

$$NNT = 1/[BR \times (1-RR)], \text{ where BR is baseline risk and RR is 0.85}$$

If the summary effect measure is odds ratio (OR), then the following formula is required:

$$NNT = [(1 - BR) + (OR \times BR)]/[BR \times (1 - OR) \times (1 - BR)]$$

Based on *BMJ* 2001; **322**: 329–33.

How are NNTs generated from relative summary effects provided by reviews? A precondition is that the relative effects are in fact consistent across studies with varying baseline risks. Empirical evidence suggests that summary RR and ORs from meta-analysis using a random effects model are reasonably constant across various baseline risks. We can explore this phenomenon in our review by subgroup meta-analysis of studies stratified according to the prognostic category of the recruited patients. When such an analysis shows consistency in relative effects, we may use them to generate NNTs. We will of course need information on our patient's clinical condition and prognosis, which may require us to draw on evidence outside our effectiveness review. We might find that the evidence of the review moderated by the patient's specific circumstances might lead to different applications in different patients. For example, considering the variation in NNTs among the risk groups outlined in Box 5.4, we might decide to treat Doppler-positive women but not Doppler-negative women among the clinically moderate risk group.

   We consider the implications of individualizing summary effects from reviews to clinical scenarios using our earlier example of antibiotic treatment in children with otitis media (Box 5.2). At an OR of 0.57, antibiotics (compared with no treatment) will reduce pain at 2–7 days among children at moderate risk of this symptom from 26% to 16.7%. This translates into 93 fewer children with pain per 1000 cases treated or an NNT of 11. This beneficial effect has to be balanced against the adverse effects that antibiotics can induce, like vomiting, diarrhoea and rash. Among children without antibiotics where only few suffer these symptoms (e.g. 10 in 1000 children, 1%), antibiotics lead to adverse effects in 9 more children per 1000 treated cases, at an OR of 1.94. This corresponds to an NNH of 111. The situation is altogether different if the baseline risk for adverse effects is high, say 300 in 1000 children, 30%. Here, an additional 154 children among 1000 treated cases will experience adverse effects. The corresponding NNH will be just 6. Judicious interpretation of findings of systematic reviews in different contexts is required to reach sound resolutions of scenarios.

> An **adverse effect** is an undesirable and unintended harmful or unpleasant reaction resulting from an *intervention*.

5.4 Generating recommendations

The usefulness of a review can be greatly enhanced by providing evidence-based 'bottom line' messages to healthcare practitioners. Generating graded practice recommendations from the findings of the studies summarized in a review helps to achieve this objective. This approach is commonly used in clinical practice guidelines. There is considerable scope for confusion when moving from evidence synthesis to recommendations. In this section we straighten out some common misconceptions and give a brief outline of the key factors to consider when generating recommendations for practice.

   Recommendations should convey a clear message and should be as simple as possible to follow in practice. To achieve this, guideline developers need to start with high quality reviews. This is the starting point for the development of recommendations

> **Evidence-based medicine** (EBM) is the conscientious, explicit and judicious use of current best evidence in making decisions about healthcare.

for action in healthcare. What we and other practitioners really want to know about recommendations is how credible they are. By credibility most people mean the trustworthiness and the reliability of a message. Credibility of a recommendation depends only in part on the strength of evidence collated from the review. Guideline developers need to make additional judgments on issues such as those listed in Box 5.5. Credibility requires that all judgements involved in a recommendation are made explicit. The criteria outlined in Box 5.5 provide one approach to explicitness in

---

Box 5.5 Key considerations when generating recommendations

Consideration

1. **Balance between desirable and undesirable effects**	Large difference between desirable and undesirable effects increases the chances of a strong recommendation. A small difference increases the likelihood of a weak recommendation.
2. **Overall strength of evidence across all critical outcomes** (see Box 5.1)	The higher the level of strength of the evidence, the higher the likelihood of a strong recommendation.
3. **Values and preferences**	Large variation in values and preferences, or great uncertainty in values and preferences, increase the likelihood of a weak recommendation.
4. **Costs (resource allocation)**	The higher the costs of an intervention, the lower the likelihood of a strong recommendation.

The implications of strong and weak recommendations

Implications	Strong recommendation	Weak recommendation
...for patients	Most patients in this situation would want the recommended course of action and only a small proportion would not.	Most people in this situation would want the recommended course of action, but many would not.
... for clinicians	Most patients should receive the recommended course of action.	Different choices will be appropriate for different patients, and the clinician must help each patient to arrive at a management decision consistent with the patient's values and preferences.
... for policy makers	The recommendation can be adopted as a policy in most situations.	Policy making will require substantial debate and involvement of many stakeholders.

classifying recommendations as strong and weak. Needless to say, strong and weak recommendations can be in favour of or against a healthcare intervention.

Recommendations are used by different groups such as healthcare professionals, patients and the general public, and local, regional or national policy makers. A strong or weak recommendation is likely to have different implications for each type of user. Healthcare professionals may interpret a strong recommendation as a directive advising them that almost all patients should receive the suggested action, and they may advise their patients accordingly. For patients, a strong recommendation may indicate that, when fully informed, most are very likely to make the same choice. Healthcare policy makers and funders may conclude from a strong recommendation that compliance with the suggested action could serve as a quality indicator to measure the performance of the organizations they commission to provide services.

A weak recommendation, on the other hand, may imply for clinicians that patients may vary in their values and preferences and as a result may take different courses of actions despite the same evidence. In this situation, clinicians may therefore advise their patients to select a treatment that best suits their personal values. For patients, a weak recommendation may imply that a considerable proportion of patients would differ in their treatment choices. They might want to clarify their own preferences in this situation. Health policy makers may conclude from weak recommendations that compliance with suggested action will not be suitable as a quality indicator. In this scenario, a documented discussion with the patient on alternative treatment options would be a better standard of care criterion.

When assigning a strong or weak grade to a recommendation, four key factors need be taken into consideration (Box 5.5). First, the balance between desirable and undesirable effects of an intervention, between its benefits and harms. For example, the proven benefit of aspirin after a heart attack to prevent a re-infarction outweighs by far the potential adverse effects and cost for the patient. This unambiguous benefit of aspirin following a myocardial infarction calls for a strong recommendation. If the benefit is less obvious or the harm to the patients, including cost and inconvenience, is more substantial, it is better that the guideline group gives a weak recommendation, implying that patients might consider alternative options and clinicians should dedicate some time eliciting the treatment options that are most in line with a patient's preferences.

The second factor is the overall strength of the evidence that confirmed the beneficial effects. Strong evidence is much more likely to result in a strong recommendation than treatment effects observed in studies of low or even very low evidence. While high quality randomized trials have demonstrated the benefit of calcium-channel blockers *versus* placebo in lowering events from coronary heart disease and from stroke, backing a strong recommendation, only case series have examined the utility of oral nifedipine for the treatment of chronic anal fissure, making strong recommendations much less likely.

The third factor is the values and preferences that patients relate to the intervention. Consider the situation of young women with newly diagnosed breast cancer. When faced with the decision, almost all will place a higher value on the life-prolonging effects of aggressive chemotherapy over treatment toxicity. Therefore, this treatment option deserves a strong recommendation. Compare this to the situation where women with advanced age have been diagnosed with breast cancer. Their decisions on aggressive chemotherapy are likely to vary and a considerable minority might place a higher value on avoiding treatment toxicity compared to the life-prolonging effects of aggressive chemotherapy. In this situation, a weak treatment recommendation appropriately reflects those distinct value judgements of the women.

The fourth factor that influences the grading of a recommendation refers to the resource use that results from a recommendation, in particular (but not exclusively) cost. Although all recommendations have implications for resource use, many groups omit an explicit consideration of this factor in their decision. Despite being more effective, the high cost of rasburicase compared to allopurinol in tumour lysis syndrome is likely to attenuate the grade of a recommendation, while the low cost of aspirin is unlikely to impair the grade of a recommendation in patients after myocardial infarction.

Summary of Step 5: Interpreting the findings

Key points about appraising review articles
- Are data on all critical and important outcomes reported?
- What is the level of strength of the evidence for each outcome?
- If the evidence in the review is trustworthy, what is its meaning for clinical practice?
- Are the recommendations derived judiciously?
- The article may not provide much of the analysis required for recommendations, but following the advice given in this Step, we might be able to generate clinically meaningful inferences for ourselves.

Key points about conducting reviews
- Set out the main findings for each critical and important outcome separately.
- Ascertain that the key points about appraising reviews listed at the end of each of the four Steps so far have been met.

- Assign a level of strength to the evidence for each outcome considering at least study design, methodological quality, consistency of results from study to study, precision of observed effect, and risk of publication and related biases.
- Explore variations in the relative effects and their reasons, particularly if the relative effects vary with baseline risk level or severity of disease. The intervention may be effective only in certain clinical groups.
- Compute the predicted absolute effects (numbers needed to treat, NNTs) according to disease severity. This way we will be able to individualize the effects observed in the review to the requirements of our patients.
- Any recommendations should be graded strong or weak considering the balance between desirable and undesirable effects, the strength of evidence across all critical and important outcomes, patients' values and preferences, and costs.

Section B: *Case studies*

The application of review theory covered in the preceding section is illustrated through the following case studies. Some readers may prefer to assimilate the review theory first before turning to the case studies. Others may read them in conjunction with the information contained in the previous section. Each case consists of a scenario requiring evidence from reviews, a demonstration of some review methods and a proposed resolution of the scenario. The interpretations of the evidence are based on specific scenarios. Judicious interpretation of findings of systematic reviews in other scenarios may lead to different resolutions. Insight into critical appraisal and conduct of a systematic review can be gained by working through the case studies.

Case study 1: Identifying and appraising systematic reviews

Case study 2: Reviewing evidence on safety of a public health intervention

Case study 3: Reviewing evidence on effectiveness of therapy

Case study 4: Reviewing evidence on accuracy of a test

Case study 5: Reviewing qualitative evidence to evaluate patient experience

Case study 6: Reviewing evidence on the effects of educational intervention

Case study 7: Gauging strength of evidence to guide decision making

Case study 8: To use or not to use a therapy? Incorporating evidence on adverse effects

● Case study 1:
Identifying and appraising systematic reviews

What is involved in identification, appraisal and application of evidence summarized in reviews?

Framing questions
↓
Identifying relevant reviews
↓
Assessing quality of the review and its evidence
↓
Summarizing the evidence
↓
Interpreting the finding

When seeking evidence from reviews to guide our clinical practice, we may face some difficulty in formulating questions. This is often due to the tension between addressing questions with either a wide or a narrow focus. Practitioners think broadly about clinical topics before making a decision for a specific patient or problem but evidence is not always summarized in this way. Nowadays we are likely to find several reviews on a question and awareness about variation in their focus is important.

This case study will demonstrate advantages and disadvantages of broad and narrow types of questions, and how to identify and appraise existing reviews. It will help us develop an approach to selecting relevant reviews when several reviews are available on a topic. It will draw on the key points about appraisal (shown at the end of each step in Section A) to make our reading of reviews more efficient.

Scenario: Drug treatment for recent onset schizophrenia

You are a psychiatrist due to see a 25-year-old amateur guitar player who has a recent diagnosis of schizophrenia. This is a mental condition where the patient may suffer symptoms such as hallucinations (often hearing voices) and delusions (unshakeable beliefs that are contrary to a person's social and cultural background), called 'positive' symptoms. There may also be emotional numbness, lack of motivation, muddled speech and thoughts, which are called 'negative' symptoms. You want to consider the available options for this patient, taking account of her preferences. Playing music is the joy of her life; thus you are aware of the importance of avoiding treatments associated with movement disorders so that your patient's guitar playing is not impaired.

Being a specialist, you are well aware of the various treatment options. These include the classical drugs such as chlorpromazine and haloperidol, and a whole range of new antipsychotic drugs. The beneficial and harmful effects of these drugs are varied. New drugs are also more expensive. Given these variations, you had been thinking about examining the literature to check whether your prescribing practice was in line with the best evidence.

This case study was developed as a learning aid in 2002. It has been retained in the second edition of this book in its original form. The results of the literature searches, therefore, are not current.

Free form question: It describes the query for which you seek an answer through a review in simple language (however vague).

Structured question: Reviewers convert free form questions into a clear and explicit format using a structured approach (see Box 1.2). This makes the query potentially answerable through existing relevant studies.

Step 1: Framing the question

Free form question

For adults with recent onset schizophrenia, what is the effectiveness of the various drug treatments and what are their harmful effects?

Structured question

The populations   Adults with recent onset schizophrenia (in this case study you are not interested in patients with unresponsive schizophrenia).

The interventions   Antipsychotic drugs, both classical and new.

The outcomes   Beneficial: improvements on 'positive' and 'negative' symptoms. This may involve psychological measurements of global or mental state of the patient.
Adverse effects: movement disorders and other side effects, e.g. somnolence.

The study design   Beneficial outcomes: review(s) of experimental studies addressing effectiveness.
Adverse effects: review(s) of experimental and observational studies addressing safety.

The question formulated above is a broad one. Of the various components of the question, the *population* is quite focused, the *interventions* and *outcomes* are broad and so are the *study designs*. Both classical and new *interventions* (of which there are more than a dozen drug treatments), both beneficial *outcomes* and adverse effects, and both experimental and observational *designs* (Box 1.4) are to be considered. You expect to find a number of reviews, which have taken a narrower focus, e.g. comparing one drug *versus* another without regard for other available options. However, this would not be suitable for your case scenario. You want to choose a treatment for your patient with the optimum balance between beneficial and adverse effects after considering all available options.

Step 2: Identifying relevant reviews

The number of reviews has increased exponentially in recent years. When searching for reviews to guide your practice, sometimes you may be faced with numerous reviews collating the findings of several studies on your topic of interest. Although this might fill you with enthusiasm, at the same time multiplicity of reviews presents a challenge. Identifying which reviews to read and which not to, may not be easy.

The Cochrane Library search

Having framed your question you decide to search the Cochrane Library. It has several databases, some of which are shown in

Effectiveness is the extent to which an *intervention* produces beneficial *outcomes* under ordinary day-to-day circumstances.

Question components

The population: A clinically suitable sample of patients.

The interventions: Comparison of groups with and without the intervention.

The outcomes: Changes in health status due to interventions.

The study design: Ways of conducting research to assess the effects of interventions.

Adverse effect is an undesirable and unintended harmful or unpleasant reaction resulting from an *intervention*.

Effect is a measure of association between an *intervention* and an *outcome*.

Box 0.1. It is the best source of reviews and protocols of reviews about effectiveness of interventions, which are included in its Cochrane Database of Systematic Reviews (CDSR). It also provides abstracts of quality assessed systematic reviews from a wide range of sources in the Database of Abstracts of Reviews of Effectiveness (DARE), and abstracts of technology assessments from a network of agencies in the Health Technology Assessment (HTA) Database. In the fourth issue of the 2009 Cochrane Library there are:

- 1906 complete reviews
- 4027 protocols of reviews
- 11 447 abstracts of quality assessed reviews
- 7596 abstracts of technology assessments.

There are several ways to find reviews in the Cochrane Library. Just by typing the words 'schizophrenia AND antipsychotics' in the query box of the 2002 Cochrane Library (Issue 3) and clicking the search button, there were 59 hits (50 reviews and 9 protocols) in CDSR and 14 hits in DARE (Box C1.1). In addition, there were three hits in the HTA Database. CDSR had several reviews, but they appeared to address very focused questions, much narrower than the question you had formulated. However, among the 14 DARE abstracts, the first three titles appeared to address a broad question similar to the one you are trying to answer. One of the HTA Database titles was relevant and it was the same as one of the three identified in DARE (Drug treatments for schizophrenia). For busy clinicians the most useful property of the DARE database is that assessment of the review's quality has already been carried out by trained staff who write the structured abstracts for this database. This may help you to decide which reviews to read in detail and, more importantly, which not to (Box C1.1).

Selecting a review to read in detail

From the titles of the DARE abstracts, it was clear to you that only three reviews have a broad focus compatible with your question. The key findings of the DARE abstracts concerning quality of their literature searches are provided in Box C1.1. The review in the *BMJ* searched comprehensively (though it reported unclearly about use of language restrictions) but it was not up-to-date. The other review in the *Annals of Pharmacotherapy* searched only one database; it used language restrictions in study selection and it was not up-to-date either.

The remaining review turned out to be a 'review of Cochrane reviews' which are not up-to-date either (last updated in 1999). Its abstracts in the DARE and HTA Databases provided a web link to its full report (www.york.ac.uk/inst/crd/EHC/ehc56.pdf). The report actually warned readers that its contents were likely to be valid for around one year following publication, by which time significant new research evidence was expected to become available. It also said that the review will be updated as part of the work for a

A **Cochrane review** is a systematic review undertaken following the methodology of the Cochrane Collaboration and is included in the Cochrane Database of Systematic reviews in the Cochrane Library.

Box C1.1 Searching the Cochrane Library for systematic reviews on drug treatment for schizophrenia and selecting a review to read in detail

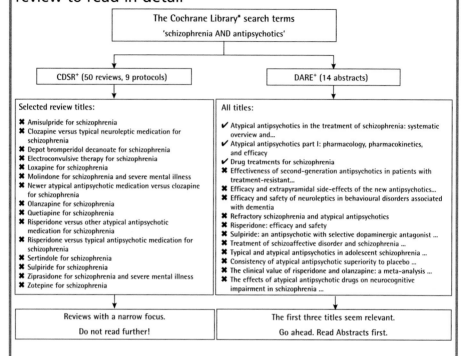

The Cochrane Library* search terms

'schizophrenia AND antipsychotics'

CDSR⁺ (50 reviews, 9 protocols)

DARE⁺ (14 abstracts)

Selected review titles:

✖ Amisulpride for schizophrenia
✖ Clozapine versus typical neuroleptic medication for schizophrenia
✖ Depot bromperidol decanoate for schizophrenia
✖ Electroconvulsive therapy for schizophrenia
✖ Loxapine for schizophrenia
✖ Molindone for schizophrenia and severe mental illness
✖ Newer atypical antipsychotic medication versus clozapine for schizophrenia
✖ Olanzapine for schizophrenia
✖ Quetiapine for schizophrenia
✖ Risperidone versus other atypical antipsychotic medication for schizophrenia
✖ Risperidone versus typical antipsychotic medication for schizophrenia
✖ Sertindole for schizophrenia
✖ Sulpiride for schizophrenia
✖ Ziprasidone for schizophrenia and severe mental illness
✖ Zotepine for schizophrenia

All titles:

✔ Atypical antipsychotics in the treatment of schizophrenia: systematic overview and...
✔ Atypical antipsychotics part I: pharmacology, pharmacokinetics, and efficacy
✔ Drug treatments for schizophrenia
✖ Effectiveness of second-generation antipsychotics in patients with treatment–resistant...
✖ Efficacy and extrapyramidal side-effects of the new antipsychotics...
✖ Efficacy and safety of neuroleptics in behavioural disorders associated with dementia
✖ Refractory schizophrenia and atypical antipsychotics
✖ Risperidone: efficacy and safety
✖ Sulpiride: an antipsychotic with selective dopaminergic antagonist ...
✖ Treatment of schizoaffective disorder and schizophrenia ...
✖ Typical and atypical antipsychotics in adolescent schizophrenia ...
✖ Consistency of atypical antipsychotic superiority to placebo ...
✖ The clinical value of risperidone and olanzapine: a meta-analysis ...
✖ The effects of atypical antipsychotic drugs on neurocognitive impairment in schizophrenia ...

Reviews with a narrow focus.

Do not read further!

The first three titles seem relevant.

Go ahead. Read Abstracts first.

Selecting a review to read in detail

Review behind DARE Abstract	Quality of its search	Decision to read further
Atypical antipsychotics in the treatment of schizophrenia: systematic overview and meta-regression analysis. *BMJ* 2000; **321**: 1371–6.	MEDLINE, EMBASE, PsycLIT and the Cochrane Controlled Trials Register searched to December 1998. No description of language restrictions.	No, do not read further. Outdated.
Atypical antipsychotics part I: pharmacology, pharmacokinetics, and efficacy. *Ann Pharmacother* 1999; **33**: 73–85.	MEDLINE only searched from July 1986 to June 1998. Study selection restricted to English language only.	No, do not read further. Outdated
Drug treatments for schizophrenia. *Effective Health Care Bull* 1999: **5(6)**. (www.york.ac.uk/inst/crd/EHC/ehc56.pdf)	Review of Cochrane reviews in the Cochrane Library 1999.	Yes. The bulletin available on the internet indicates that an update has been commissioned. Obtain the most up-to-date review from www.ncchta.org/project/htapubs.asp

* *Search results from the Cochrane Library 2002, Issue 3*
⁺ *CDSR, the Cochrane Database of Systematic Reviews; DARE, the Database of Abstracts of Reviews of Effectiveness (see Box 0.1 for details).*

forthcoming report commissioned by the UK National Health Service HTA Programme.

This information led you to check the web pages of the HTA programme (Box 0.1). The above project had been superseded by a similar one commissioned by the HTA programme and data had recently been published (but it was not yet included in the Cochrane Library's HTA database). This review, it turned out, included no less than eight systematic reviews addressing benefits, adverse effects and cost-effectiveness of new antipsychotics, including amisulpride, clozapine, olanzapine, quetiapine, risperidone, sertindole, ziprasidone and zotepine. Given the fact that clozapine is a relatively old drug that was reintroduced for treating those with unresponsive schizophrenia, you leave it out of the rest of this case study. The reviews were actually based on updates of the Cochrane reviews that you had already identified in CDSR. This search emphasizes the importance of checking if reviews have already been done or are in progress before even considering preparing a new systematic review.

Step 3: Assessing quality of the review

Given the large size of this report, and the fact that the included reviews had been prepared using the same protocols, you can take a two-step approach to their appraisal. First, check the quality of the overall report, and if satisfactory, then take a closer look at the amount and quality of the evidence included in each of the reviews when interpreting the findings.

In this report the Cochrane reviews from 1999 had been updated with relevant studies found in comprehensive literature searches of more than 20 databases, 10 conference proceedings, ongoing trials registers, scanning of the reference lists of retrieved papers and reports of studies submitted by the companies which produced the drugs. In addition, further searches had been carried out for non-randomized studies of rare or long-term harmful outcomes. The quality of the included evidence was assessed by using separate checklists for effectiveness and safety studies. The studies were synthesized and interpreted in an appropriate way. Although assessment for the risk of publication and related biases had been limited because of scarcity of suitable data, the searches had been comprehensive enough to reassure you that this report provided the best available information (Box C1.2).

Safety relates to adverse effects associated with *interventions*.

Step 4: Summarizing the evidence

There were 171 experimental studies and 52 observational studies addressing rare or long-term effects in the review. However, the quality of the studies was not always ideal and the number of head-to-head comparisons evaluating similar outcomes was

Box C1.2 Appraising the overall quality of a Health Technology Assessment report on systematic reviews of drug treatment for schizophrenia

Step 1: Framing questions
- The report is based on predefined questions.
- The questions were modified during the review, but justifications were provided.
- The questions do not seem to have been unduly influenced by knowledge of the results of studies.

Step 2: Identifying relevant literature
- The searches appear to be comprehensive. Over 20 databases, 10 conference proceedings, ongoing trials registers and the reference lists of retrieved papers have been searched. In addition, the companies that produce the drugs have submitted reports of their own studies.
- The selection criteria were set *a priori* and applied by two reviewers independently.
- It seems unlikely that relevant studies might have been missed.

Step 3: Assessing quality of the literature
- Quality assessment has been undertaken for studies included in the review.
- Quality has been used as a criterion for study selection (Step 2): for effectiveness experimental studies were included and for safety clear inclusion criteria concerning study designs were formulated.
- A more detailed quality assessment of selected studies has been carried out. The quality items seem to be appropriate for the question.
- Variation in quality has been explored as an explanation for heterogeneity and meta-analysis seems to have been used selectively where appropriate (Step 4).

Step 4: Summarizing the evidence
- Heterogeneity of effects has been evaluated.
- The exploration for heterogeneity was planned in advance in broad terms and with variations within the included systematic reviews.
- Variation in studies' clinical characteristics has been found to be an explanation for heterogeneity.
- Variation in study design and quality has also been found to be an explanation for heterogeneity.
- Meta-analysis seems to have been used selectively and appropriately in the light of information gathered on heterogeneity and its reasons.

Step 5: Interpreting the findings
- Risk of publication and related biases has been addressed in a limited way because suitable data were not available for all outcomes.
- There is no formal categorization of strength of inferences according to quality of evidence, but the conclusions are clearly made with consideration of the quality of most studies.
- The credibility or trustworthiness of the evidence included in the review – the quality of included studies is limited and so is the number of relevant comparisons.

> • The meaning of the review's findings for clinical practice – the review provides information that has limitations which make it difficult to generate durable inferences for practice.
>
> *Critical appraisal based on key points listed at the end of each step in Section A of this book*
> *The full review report is available from www.ncchta.org/project/htapubs.asp.*

limited. An overview of the findings of the various reviews is provided in Box C1.3. The new drugs most frequently assessed for their effectiveness and safety were olanzapine and risperidone.

Beneficial effects

Evidence suggested that both classical and new antipsychotics had comparable levels of effectiveness. There were no clear differences in effectiveness between the various new antipsychotics. No single new antipsychotic agent stood out as being more effective than any of the others, nor did they collectively seem to be superior to classical drugs.

Adverse effects

The new antipsychotics possibly had fewer adverse effects in terms of movement disorders than the classical drug haloperidol. For example, risperidone showed a relative risk (RR) of 0.64 (95% CI 0.56–0.73) for 'movement disorders' based on seven studies. The new agents all seemed to have slightly different side-effects from haloperidol, and these may vary in importance to those with schizophrenia and their carers.

Daytime sleepiness (somnolence) and drowsiness possibly occurred more frequently in those given clozapine or quetiapine than in those given classical drugs. Olanzapine, amisulpride, sertindole and perhaps risperidone may cause less somnolence than classical drugs. There was no evidence to suggest that the other new drugs were any more or less sedating than the classical drugs.

Step 5 Interpreting the findings

It is important to assess the strength of evidence when interpreting the findings using the key points from Step 5. The available evidence for the effectiveness and safety of the new antipsychotics compared to classical drugs was, in general, of low quality and it was often based on short-term studies. The basis for choosing between the classical and the newer drugs was not as strong as one would like. However, for olanzapine and risperidone there was the largest body of evidence and it suggested effectiveness comparable or better than classical drugs and similar to other new drugs. The evidence showed significantly less adverse effects such as movement disorders and somnolence. Although

Strength of evidence describes the extent to which we can be confident that the estimate of an observed effect is correct for important questions. It takes into account directness of outcome measure, study design, study quality, heterogeneity, imprecision and publication bias (this is not an exhaustive list).

Box C1.3 Assessing the quality of evidence included in systematic reviews of drug treatment for schizophrenia in a Health Technology Assessment report

	Total number of experimental studies		Effectiveness (alleviation of schizophrenic symptoms)		Safety (movement disorders and somnolence/drowsiness)	
	vs classical drugs	vs other new drugs	vs classical drugs	vs other new drugs	vs classical drugs	vs other new drugs
Amisulpride	13	4	Marginally better on most outcomes	No important differences	Less movement disorders	Few data, no clear differences
Olanzapine	24	14	Mostly marginally better	No important differences	Less movement disorders, less drowsiness	No clear differences
Quetiapine	9	1	Better on most outcomes, often marginally	Only one comparison available	Less movement disorders, may cause sleepiness	Very few data available
Risperidone	27	19	Better on most outcomes, often marginally	No important differences	Less movement disorders, less somnolence	Similar
Sertindole	2	0	No clear differences, few data	No comparisons available	Less movement disorders	
Ziprasidone	9	4	Few data in public domain*	Studies not in public domain*	Less movement disorders than haloperidol	Data not publicly available*
Zotepine	8	3	Equal or better results	Very few comparisons available	Less movement disorders, no differences for somnolence	Very few data available

The full review report is available from www.hta.nhsweb.nhs.uk/

*One governing body (UK National Institute for Clinical Excellence – www.nice.org.uk/cat.asp?e=32878), after considering this evidence, concluded that for patients with newly diagnosed schizophrenia, prescribing one of the following newer oral antipsychotic drugs should be considered: amisulpride, olanzapine, quetiapine, risperidone or zotepine. In drawing its conclusion, the governing body had access to confidential information which is not available in the public domain. Its recommendation is said to have a time limit of 3 years, after which it is likely to be reviewed again, taking into account the newly accumulated evidence.

the quality of the evidence was variable, when subgroup analysis was carried out on the highest quality studies available, results remained unchanged. Having considered the evidence yourself, you were more confident to use olanzapine or risperidone unless there were clear contraindications.

Resolution of scenario

Given the musical interest of your patient, you felt that a therapeutic choice based on avoiding movement disorders and somnolence made sense as it would not interfere with her guitar playing. You decide to commence either olanzapine or risperidone with careful monitoring of the beneficial and adverse effects. If the treatment is not effective in alleviating symptoms or if there are unacceptable side-effects, you will switch to the other drug.

● Case study 2:
Reviewing evidence on safety of a public health intervention

Step 1
Framing questions
↓
Step 2
Identifying relevant literature
↓
Step 3
Assessing quality of the literature
↓
Step 4
Summarizing the evidence
↓
Step 5
Interpreting the findings

Reviews of safety of interventions are not as common as those of their effectiveness. Research on safety may relate to common harmful outcomes, which may be captured in the same studies that address effectiveness. However, most experimental studies focus primarily on effectiveness and secondarily on safety – any information on safety is often only a by-product. Harmful outcomes can be rare and they may develop over a long time. There are considerable difficulties in designing and conducting safety studies to capture these outcomes, as a large number of people need to be observed over a long period of time. In this situation, observational, not experimental, studies are needed. With this background, systematic reviews on safety have to include evidence from studies with a range of designs.

This case study demonstrates how to seek and assess evidence on safety using a published review of a preventive public health intervention. This topic is important because public health interventions have an impact on large groups of populations and it has to be assured that the benefit outweighs any potential harm. This case study provides a demonstration of the application of review theory related to question formulation, literature identification and quality assessment of studies on safety. It was developed as a learning aid in 2002. For the second edition of this book, we searched the literature for reviews published since the year 2000. There were 9 reviews which evaluated whether it was safe to provide population-wide drinking water fluoridation. Findings of all new reviews were compatible with the conclusions of the original case study. So we decided to keep this case study on safety in the same form as it was presented in the first edition.

Safety relates to adverse effects associated with *interventions*.

Effectiveness is the extent to which an intervention produces beneficial outcomes under ordinary day-to-day circumstances.

Scenario: Safety of public water fluoridation

You are a public health professional in a locality that has public water fluoridation. For many years, you and your colleagues have held the belief that it improves dental health. Recently your local authority has been under pressure from various interest groups to consider the safety of this public health intervention because they fear that it is causing cancer.

In the past, most public health decisions have been based on judgement and practical feasibility; however, in recent years there has been an increasing demand to examine the scientific basis behind the issues under consideration. You have been observing this development with interest and now you have the chance to apply this approach yourself. In anticipation of the discussion about the safety of water fluoridation intensifying in the near future, you want to prepare well and use evidence from the literature to inform any future decisions.

Using Medline through the freely accessible PubMed interface (www.ncbi.nlm.nih.gov/entrez/query.fcgi), you enter 'drinking water fluoridation' into the query box and find 588 citations that may potentially provide information on your issue. Although you are a bit shocked about this large number of studies and are wondering how to squeeze the necessary reading time into your already packed daily routine, you perform a PubMed Clinical Queries search (www.ncbi.nlm.nih.gov/entrez/query/static/clinical.html) using the same query in the Systematic Reviews feature. You find four citations; three are reviews and one is suitable for addressing your current concern:

- Systematic review of water fluoridation. *BMJ* 2000; **321**: 855–9. (seems relevant)
- Association of Down's syndrome and water fluoride level: a systematic review of the evidence. *BMC Public Health* 2001; **1**: 6. (does not seem directly relevant)
- Exposure to high fluoride concentrations in drinking water is associated with decreased birth rates. *J Toxicol Environ Health* 1994; **42**: 109–21. (does not seem directly relevant)
- Factors influencing the effectiveness of sealants – a meta-analysis. *Community Dent Oral Epidemiol* 1993; **21**: 261–8. (does not seem relevant)

Incidentally if you do an internet search on the same day using the Google search engine (www.google.com), you will have an overwhelming 15 100 hits, but in second position among them will be the full report of the systematic review on which the above relevant paper is based:

- A systematic review of water fluoridation. NHS Centre for Reviews and Dissemination (CRD) Report 18. York, University of York, 2000 (available at www.york.ac.uk/inst/crd/fluorid.htm)

Your impression is that using the review is the right starting point as it may save an enormous amount of time compared with obtaining and reading the large number of individual studies. (The above search was undertaken in 2002.)

Free form question: It describes the query for which you seek an answer through a review in simple language (however vague).

Structured question: Reviewers convert free form questions into a clear and explicit format using a structured approach (see Box 1.2). This makes the query potentially answerable through existing relevant studies.

Step 1: Framing the question

Free form question

Is it safe to provide population-wide drinking water fluoridation to prevent caries?

Structured questions

The populations   Populations receiving drinking water sourced through a public water supply.

The exposures   Fluoridation of drinking water (naturally or artificially) compared with non-fluoridated water.

The outcomes   Cancer is the main outcome of interest for the debate in your health authority. You also decide to consider other outcomes such as fluorosis (mottled teeth) and fractures as there has been concern about the effect of fluorides on bones.

The study designs   Comparative studies of any design (Box 1.4) examining the outcomes in at least two population groups, one with fluoridated drinking water and the other without.

The original review was conducted to address five different questions. This case study will only focus (not least for the sake of brevity and simplicity) on the question of safety related to the *outcomes* described above.

Question components

The population: A suitable sample of participants.

The exposures: Comparison of groups with and without the exposure.

The outcomes: Changes in health status due to interventions.

The study design: Ways of conducting research to assess the effect of interventions.

Step 2: Identifying relevant literature

To cast as wide a net as possible to capture as many relevant citations as possible, a wide range of medical, political and environmental/scientific databases were searched to identify primary studies of the effects of water fluoridation (Box C2.1). The range of databases searched in this review is far beyond what is usually covered in reviews of clinical questions. The electronic searches are also supplemented by hand searching Index Medicus and Excerpta Medica for several years (back to 1945) to cover the time period before Medline and Embase became accessible electronically. The search process was further supported by use of the internet. Various internet search engines were used to find web pages that might provide references. In addition, web pages were set up to inform the public about the review and to enable individuals and organizations to submit references or reports. Not surprisingly, there was a degree of duplication in the captured citations resulting from searching a wide range of databases. After the removal of duplicates, 3246 citations remained, from which the relevant studies were selected for review.

This comprehensive search of a variety of databases yielded far more citations than are commonly found when searching the literature for focused clinical questions (compare with Case study 3). The potential relevance of the identified citations was assessed – 2511 citations were found to be irrelevant. The full papers of the remaining 735 citations were assessed to select those primary studies in humans that directly related to fluoride in drinking water supplies, comparing at least two groups. These criteria excluded 481 studies, leaving 254 studies in the review. They came from 30 countries and were published in 14 languages between 1939 and 2000. Of these studies, 175 were relevant to the question of safety (Box C2.1).

Identifying relevant literature:
- Develop search term combinations
- Search relevant electronic databases
- Search other relevant resources
- Obtain full papers of potentially relevant citations
- Include/exclude studies using pre-set selection criteria

Step 3: Assessing study quality

Study design threshold for study selection

Use of *study design* as a marker for ensuring a minimum level of quality has been described as an inclusion criterion in Step 2. This approach is easier to apply when seeking evidence of effectiveness using experimental studies. This is because randomized studies are often difficult (if not impossible) to conduct at a community level for a public health intervention such as water fluoridation. Thus, systematic reviews assessing safety of such interventions have to look beyond experimental studies, and include evidence from various types of *study design*. Considering the nature of the research likely to be available to address safety issues, in this review a simple *design* threshold was used as a selection criterion: Comparative studies of any design were included, but those without any comparative information were excluded (Box 2.4). In this way studies that provided information about the harmful effects of exposure to fluoridated water compared with non-exposure were selected.

Confounding is a situation in comparative studies where the effect of an *exposure* on an *outcome* is distorted due to the association of the *outcome* with another factor, which can prevent or cause the *outcome* independent of the *exposure*. Data analysis may be adjusted for confounding in observational studies.

Quality assessment of safety studies

After selecting studies of an acceptable design, their in-depth assessment for the risk of various biases allows us to gauge the quality of the evidence in a more refined way. The objective of the included studies is to compare groups exposed to fluoridated drinking water with groups without such exposure, and look for rates of undesirable outcomes without bias. Step 3 shows how to develop and use study quality assessments in a review of effectiveness. For safety studies to have validity, they must ascertain *exposures* and *outcomes* in such a way that the risk of misclassification is minimized. They must also establish the association between *exposures* and *outcomes*, adjusting for the confounding effect of other factors. These features are likely to be more robustly implemented in experimental studies, but they

A **comparative study** is one where the effect of an exposure is assessed using comparison groups.

The **validity** of a study depends on the degree to which its design, conduct and analysis minimizes **biases**.

Bias either exaggerates or underestimates the 'true' effect of an *exposure*.

Box C2.1 Identification of relevant literature on safety of public water fluoridation

Electronic databases searched

1. Agricola
2. BIOSIS Previews (a database on life sciences)
3. CAB Health
4. CINAHL (Cumulative Index of Nursing and Allied Health Literature);
5. Conference Papers Index
6. EI Compendex (Engineering Index)
7. EMBASE (Excerpta Medica Database)
8. Enviroline
9. Food Science and Technology Abstracts (FSTA)
10. Health Service Technology, Administration and Research (Healthstar)
11. HSR Proj
12. JICST-E Plus (Japanese Science and Technology)
13. Latin American and Caribbean Health Sciences Literature (LILACS)
14. MEDLINE and OldMEDLINE
15. NTIS
16. PASCAL
17. PSYCLIT
18. Public Affairs Information Service (PAIS)
19. Science Citation Index and Social Science Citation Index
20. System for Information on Grey Literature in Europe (SIGLE)
21. TOXLINE
22. Water Resources Abstracts
23. Waternet

Study identification flow chart

Potentially relevant citations identified through comprehensive electronic searching of databases, hand searching and contact with experts

n = 3246 citations with titles and abstracts

Citations excluded
n = 2511

Retrieval of hard copies of potentially relevant citations
n = 735 papers

Studies excluded after assessment of full text
n = 481

Studies included in the original review but excluded from this case
n = 79

Studies on safety included in the published review
n = 175

Cancer: n = 26
Fluorosis: n = 88
Bone fractures: n = 29
Other adverse outcomes: n = 32

The original search is part of the full report of the review available at www.york.ac.uk/inst/crd/fluorid.htm

typically assess a relatively small number of participants over a short duration of follow-up. So in such studies there is only a limited chance of detecting rare *outcomes* that often do not follow immediately after *exposure*. Hence quality assessment has to be planned somewhat differently to that in reviews of effectiveness of interventions. In this case study the quality issues related to safety studies are briefly examined.

Anticipating that experimental studies would be scarce, reviewers planned study quality assessment based on features that would minimize biases of the various types described above. They assessed ascertainment of *exposures* and *outcomes*, i.e. how did the investigators make sure that the study participants had the *exposures* and *outcomes* under question. A prospective design would facilitate this. This means that those exposed (and unexposed) to fluoridated water and those developing cancer (and remaining free of cancer) are more likely to be correctly identified in these groups if they are assessed in a prospective fashion. The *exposure* is likely to be more accurately ascertained if the study commenced soon after water fluoridation and the *outcomes* are likely to be more accurately ascertained if the follow-up is long and if it is assessed blind to *exposure* status.

When examining how the effect of *exposure* on *outcome* was established, reviewers assessed if the comparison groups were similar in all respects other than their exposure to fluoridated water. This is because the other differences may be related to the *outcomes* of interest independent of the drinking water fluoridation, and this would bias the comparison. For example, if the people exposed to fluoridated water had other risk factors that make them more prone to cancer, the apparent association between *exposure* and *outcome* may be explained by the more frequent occurrence of these factors among the exposed groups compared with the non-exposed groups. Technically speaking, such studies suffer from confounding. In a (large) experimental study, confounding factors are expected to be approximately equally distributed between groups (but no such studies exist on water fluoridation). In observational studies their distribution may be unequal. Primary researchers can statistically adjust for these differences when estimating the effect of *exposure* on *outcomes* (using multivariable modelling). The larger the number of variables adjusted for, the more likely it is that the observed association between *exposure* and *outcome* will be 'true'.

Put simply, use of a prospective design, robust ascertainment of *exposure* and *outcomes*, and control for confounding are the generic issues one would look for in quality assessment of studies on safety. Assessing these methodological features in safety studies of water fluoridation will require development of quality criteria specific to this topic. For example, studies commencing within 1 year of water fluoridation would be able to ascertain *exposure* better than those commencing within 1–3 years, which

> **Effect** is a measure of association between an *exposure* and an *outcome*.

in turn will be better than those commencing after 3 years. This way studies would range from satisfactorily meeting quality criteria, to having some deficiencies, to not meeting the criteria at all, and they can be assigned to one of three prespecified quality categories as shown in Box C2.2.

Description of quality of the selected studies

Based on the degree to which studies comply with the quality criteria, a quality hierarchy can be developed (Box C2.2). None of the included studies is in the highest quality category, but this is because experimental studies are non-existent and control for confounding is not always ideal in observational studies (none is adjusted for three or more confounding factors in the analysis). Many studies lacked a prospective design, which makes ascertainment of *exposure* and assessment of *outcomes* difficult. More details of the study quality may be obtained from the review, but the general dearth of quality evidence in reviews of safety of interventions is not surprising to those experienced in this field.

The quality assessment for studies addressing the three harmful *outcomes* assigns low quality to the vast majority of the available evidence, only a few studies are classified as having medium quality, none has high quality (Box C2.2). Fortunately (because cancer is of major interest in this case study) studies examining the association between fluoridation and cancer show the highest quality as compared to those examining the other two harmful *outcomes* related to bones.

Step 4: Summarizing the evidence

Summarizing the evidence from studies with a large variety of designs and quality is not easy as highlighted in Steps 4 and 5. The review provides details of how the differences between study results were investigated and how they were summarized (with or without meta-analysis). This case study restricts itself to summarizing the findings narratively for the outcomes below:

Cancer

The association between exposure to fluoridated water and cancer in general was examined in 26 studies. Of these, 10 examined all-cause cancer incidence or mortality in 22 analyses. Eleven analyses found a negative association (fewer cancers due to exposure), nine found a positive association and two found no association. Only two studies found statistical significance. Thus, no clear association between water fluoridation and increased incidence or mortality was apparent. While a broad number of cancer types were represented in the included studies, bone/joint and thyroid cancers were of particular concern due to fluoride uptake by these organs. Six studies of osteosarcoma and water fluoridation reporting

Box C2.2 A quality assessment checklist for studies on safety of public water fluoridation

Quality assessment checklist

Quality issues	Quality categories	
	High* – Moderate	Low
Prospective design	Prospective	Prospective or retrospective
Exposure ascertainment	Study commenced within 3 years of water fluoridation	Study commenced after 3 years of water fluoridation
Outcome ascertainment	Long follow-up and blind assessment	Short follow-up and unblinded assessment
Control for confounding	Adjustment for at least one confounding factor	No adjustment for confounding factors

* High-quality studies were prospective, commencing within 1 year of water fluoridation, followed up people for at least 5 years, used blinding (or other robust methods) to ascertain outcomes and adjusted for at least three confounding factors (or used randomization) – no such studies existed.

Description of study quality

Information on quality presented as 100% stacked bars separately for studies evaluating different harmful outcomes. Data in the stacks represent the number of studies in moderate and low quality categories. There were no high quality studies.

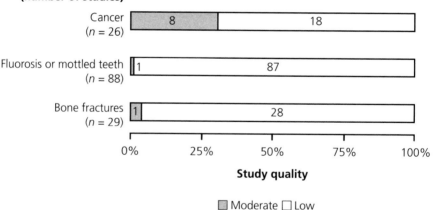

variance data found no statistically significant differences. Thyroid cancer was considered by only two studies and these also did not find a statistically significant association with water fluoride levels. Overall, from the research evidence presented, no association was detected between water fluoridation and mortality from any cancer or from bone or thyroid cancers specifically. These findings were also borne out in the moderate quality subgroup of studies.

Fluorosis

Dental flourosis is the most frequently studied harmful outcome, as reflected by the largest number (88) of studies included. Meta-regression analysis showed a strong (statistically significant) association between fluoride level and the prevalence of dental fluorosis.

Bone fractures

Twenty nine of the included studies investigated a variety of fracture sites; hip fracture was included in 18 of them. There are no definite patterns of association for any of the fractures. Similarly to the cancer studies, the studies showed similar numbers of positive and negative associations. Hip fracture analysed as a subgroup also showed no association with exposure to fluoridated drinking water.

Step 5: Interpreting the findings

In this case scenario, you focused on safety of a community-based public health intervention. The generally low quality of available studies means that interpretation must be with appropriate caution. The elaborate efforts in searching an unusually large number of databases provide some safeguard against missing relevant studies and ongoing research. The strength of the evidence summarized in this review is likely to be low, but it is as good as it is going to get in the foreseeable future.

Cancer is the *outcome* of most interest in the case scenario. No association is found between *exposure* to fluoridated water and specific cancers or all cancers. The interpretation of the results in this review may be limited because of the low quality of studies, but the findings for the cancer *outcomes* are also supported by the moderate quality studies.

Fluorosis (mottled teeth) shows a simple association and also a dose–response relationship with increasing exposure to water fluoridation. When compared with a fluoride level of 0.4 ppm (parts per million), a level of 1.0 ppm had an estimated number needed to treat (NNT) of 6 (range 4–21), sometimes called number needed to harm (NNH) in this context. This means that on average, for every six people exposed to the higher concentrations of fluorides, one additional person has mottled teeth. Bone fractures did not show an association with water fluoridation.

> The **strength of the evidence** lies in the relevance of the outcomes, the methodological quality of the included studies, the heterogeneity of results, the precision and size of effects, etc, features that underpin the trust in the inferences generated from a review.

> A dose-response relationship demonstrates that at higher doses the strength of association between exposure and outcome is increased.

Resolution of the scenario

After having spent some time reading and understanding the review, you are impressed by the sheer amount of literature relevant to the question of safety. However, you are somewhat disappointed about the poor quality of the available primary studies. Of course, examining safety only makes sense in a context where the intervention has some beneficial effect. Benefit and harm have to be compared to provide the basis for decision making. Regarding the issue of the beneficial effect of public water fluoridation, you are reassured by the review that your prior belief and that of your health authority is correct: drinking water fluoridation does prevent caries. You can now go on to evaluate the findings of the review on safety – reduction in caries by introducing fluoridation can be considered in context with cancer, fluorosis, bone fractures and other problems.

When the pressure from the interest groups raises the profile of the safety issue again, you will be able to reassure them that there is no evidence to link cancer with drinking water fluoridation. You will also be able to reassure them that there is no risk of fractures to bones. However, you will have to admit the risk of dental fluorosis, which appears to be dose dependent. Those concerned about this issue can be given advice about examining their fluoride intake from other means. You may also want to measure the fluoride concentration in your area's water supply to openly share this information with the interest groups.

Being able to quantify the safety concerns of your population through a review, albeit from studies of moderate–low quality, allows your health authority, politicians and the public to consider the balance between beneficial and adverse effects of water fluoridation. For some, the prevention of caries is of primary importance, so they would prefer fluoridation. On the other hand, aesthetic reasons may play a more important role for others who would prefer to have caries removed occasionally rather than have mottled teeth. In any case, you are able to reassure all parties that there is currently no evidence of a risk of cancer or bone fractures from drinking water fluoridation.

● Case study 3:
Reviewing evidence on effectiveness of therapy

Step 1
Framing questions
↓
Step 2
Identifying relevant literature
↓
Step 3
Assessing quality of the literature
↓
Step 4
Summarizing the evidence
↓
Step 5
Interpreting the findings

Not all reviews can provide answers that have immediate practical implications. And this may be due to a dearth of relevant studies. But lack of evidence of effectiveness should not be interpreted as evidence of lack of effectiveness.

This case study will demonstrate how to seek and assess evidence of therapeutic effectiveness in a review and how to act when faced with limited evidence. Based on a published review, it will provide a good demonstration of the application of review theory related to literature identification, study quality assessment and synthesis without meta-analysis.

Scenario: Antimicrobial therapy for chronic wounds

You are a clinical research fellow in an academic primary healthcare practice. There are a large number of patients with chronic wounds of various aetiologies. You have taken it upon yourself to develop an evidence-based clinical strategy for use of antimicrobials in management of these patients. Your initial discussions with other members of the practice reveal that they base their management on:

- what they had learnt many years ago during medical school
- what they observed from the nurses on the wards during postgraduate training
- what they have been told by pharmaceutical company representatives.

Hardly anybody could underpin their advice by good evidence. There are a variety of antimicrobial products and there seems to be no clear way forward.

You are keen to conduct a review yourself but, sensibly, you first decide to see if there is one already out there in the literature. You search MEDLINE using PubMed Clinical Queries at www.ncbi.nlm. nih.gov/entrez/query/static/clinical.html. You type 'antimicrobial chronic wounds' in the query box of the Systematic Reviews feature and click the Go button. You find the following references, which are two reports of a relevant review:

- Systematic review of antimicrobial agents used for chronic wounds. *Br J Surgery* 2001; **88**: 4–21. (this review is based on the citation below).
- Systematic review of wound care management: (3) antimicrobial

agents for chronic wounds. *Health Technol Assess* 2000: **4**; 21. (available at www.ncchta.org/execsumm/summ421.htm).

This case study was developed as a learning aid in 2002. An update search carried out for the second edition of this book revealed one further review:

- Antibiotics and antiseptics for venous leg ulcers. *Cochrane Database Syst Rev* 2008; Issue 1: CD003557.

Its findings were compatible with the conclusions of the original case study. So we decided to keep this case study on safety in the same form as it was presented in the first edition. In the section on resolution of scenario we provide additional information from this new review.

Step 1: Framing the question

Free form question

Which of the many available antimicrobial products improve healing in patients with chronic wounds?

Structured question (also see Boxes 1.2 and 1.3)

The population	Adults with various forms of chronic wounds being cared for in an ambulatory setting. We narrow down the definition of chronic wounds to diabetic ulcer, venous ulcer, pressure ulcer and chronic ulcer (excluding pilonidal sinus – which was included in the related reviews – from further consideration in this case study).
The interventions	Systemic or topical antimicrobial preparations (e.g. antibiotics, antifungal, antiviral, antiseptic agents) compared with usual treatment, placebo or alternative antimicrobial products (excluding studies about prevention).
The outcomes	A range of assessment for wound healing, e.g. complete healing, change in ulcer size, rate of healing, time to heal, etc. Complete wound healing is the clinically relevant outcome while the rest are surrogates.
The study designs	Comparative studies with or without randomization (selection of non-randomized studies restricted to those with a concurrent control group).

Question components

The population: A clinically suitable sample of patients.

The interventions: Comparison of groups with and without the intervention.

The outcomes: Changes in health status due to interventions.

The study design: Ways of conducting research to assess the effect of interventions.

Surrogate *outcome* measurements substitute for direct outcome measures. They include physiological variables or measures of subclinical disease. To be valid, the surrogate must be statistically correlated with the clinically relevant outcome.

Step 2: Identifying relevant literature

A comprehensive search was undertaken by the reviewers (without language restrictions) to identify as many relevant published and unpublished studies as possible. The electronic search covered 17 databases from their inception to January 2000 (Box C3.1). The combination of search terms used for the Medline database is shown in Box C3.2. Other databases were searched using a modified combination of these terms. In addition, manual searches of five relevant journals not covered by the electronic databases, 12 proceedings of relevant meetings and bibliographies of all retrieved articles were undertaken. A panel of subject experts was also consulted to identify studies not captured by the searches. Examples of going to such great lengths to hunt down relevant literature are not as common as one might think in the field of systematic reviews. The initial search provides 400 possibly relevant citations. After screening their titles and abstracts, 150 papers are retrieved for examination of the full text. Despite the exhaustive efforts, ultimately only 22 studies (including over 1000 patients) are found that address the question posed.

> **Identifying relevant literature**
> - Develop search term combinations
> - Search relevant electronic databases
> - Search other relevant resources
> - Select citations to retrieve potentially relevant papers
> - Include/exclude studies using pre-set selection criteria

Step 3: Assessing study quality

Study design threshold for study selection

From the outset, there was a worry that only a few studies with sound designs would be available. So the threshold for study selection had been lowered to allow observational studies with concurrent controls to be included along with randomized controlled trials and experimental studies without randomization (Box 1.4). Comparative studies with historical controls and case-control studies were excluded because of the higher risk of bias associated with these designs (Box 2.4). Of the 22 studies selected, 18 claimed to be experimental studies (but only four were clearly randomized, though with some deficiencies in concealment of allocation), and four were observational cohort studies with concurrent controls.

> **Study design filter** employs a search term combination to capture citations of studies of a particular design.

Description of quality of the selected studies

The development of a quality checklist is outlined in Box C3.2. The selected studies are systematically examined for key generic biases: Is there potential for selection bias?, for performance bias?, for measurement bias? or for attrition bias? (Box 3.2). At the same time, quality issues specific to the *populations*, *interventions* and *outcomes* of the review question were considered. In this review, appropriateness of inclusion and exclusion criteria and

> **Bias** either exaggerates or underestimates the 'true' effect of an *intervention*.

> The **quality** of a study depends on the degree to which its design, conduct and analysis minimizes **biases**.

Box C3.1 Identification of relevant literature on antimicrobials for chronic wounds

Electronic databases searched*

1. BIOSIS Previews (a database on life sciences)
2. British Diabetic Association Database
3. CINAHL (Cumulative Index of Nursing and Allied Health Literature)
4. CISCOM (Computerised Information Service for Complementary Medicine)
5. Cochrane Database of Systematic Reviews (CDSR)
6. Cochrane Wounds Groups developing database
7. Current Research in Britain (CRIB)
8. Database of Abstracts of Reviews of Effectiveness (DARE)
9. DHSS (Database produced by the Department of Health, UK on health services provided by the NHS nursing and primary care; people with disabilities and elderly people)
10. Dissertation Abstracts
11. EMBASE (Excerpta Medica Database)
12. Index to Scientific and Technological Proceedings
13. ISI® Science Citation Index
14. MEDLINE (see search term combinations in Box C3.2)
15. National Research Register (NRR)
16. Royal College of Nursing Database
17. System for Information on Grey Literature in Europe (SIGLE)

Study identification flow chart

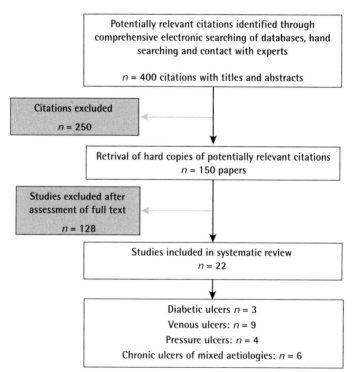

Potentially relevant citations identified through comprehensive electronic searching of databases, hand searching and contact with experts

n = 400 citations with titles and abstracts

Citations excluded
n = 250

Retrival of hard copies of potentially relevant citations
n = 150 papers

Studies excluded after assessment of full text
n = 128

Studies included in systematic review
n = 22

Diabetic ulcers *n* = 3
Venous ulcers: *n* = 9
Pressure ulcers: *n* = 4
Chronic ulcers of mixed aetiologies: *n* = 6

* Economic evaluations were included in the original review, but as the question in this case study is concerned with effectiveness, we have not described them here.

Box C3.2 Search term combination for Ovid MEDLINE database to identify citations on antimicrobials for chronic wounds

The original search term combination consists of 58 sets of terms. The following table shows only a selection of these. The purpose is to demonstrate how to build a search term combination.

Question components and a selection of relevant terms	Type of terms Free	MeSH	Boolean operator (*see glossary*)
The populations: patients with various forms of chronic wounds			
1. decubitus ulcer/ or foot ulcer		x	
2. leg ulcer/ or varicose ulcer/		x	
3. skin ulcer/		x	
4. diabetic foot/		x	
5. ((plantar or diabetic or heel or venous or stasis or arterial) adj. ulcer).tw	x		OR (captures *population*)
6. ((decubitus or foot or diabetic or ischaemic or pressure) adj. ulcer).tw	x		
7. ((pressure or bed) adj. Sore$	x		
8. *additional terms (see in original report of the review)*			
9. or/1–9			
The interventions: treatments for chronic wounds			
10. debridement/ or biological dressings/ or bandages		x	
11. occlusive dressings/ or clothing/ or wound healing/		x	
12. antibiotics/ or growth substances/ or platelet-derived growth factor/		x	
13. (debridement or dressing$ or compress$ or cream$ or (growth adj factor$)).tw	x		OR (captures *intervention*)
14. antibiotic$ or (electric adj therapy) or laser$ or nutrition$ or surg$).tw	x		
15. (homeopath$ or acupuncture or massage or reflexology or ultrasound).tw	x		
16. *additional terms (see in original report of the review)*			
17. or/10–17			
The outcomes			
No search is performed to capture *outcomes*			
18. and/9,17			AND (combines *population* and *intervention*)
The study designs			
19. random allocation/ or randomized controlled trials/		x	
20. controlled clinical trials/ or clinical trials phase I/ or clinical trials phase II/		x	
21. single-blind method/ or double blind method/		x	OR (captures *study designs*)
22. ((random$ adj controlled adj trial$) or (prospective adj random$).tw.	x		
23. *additional terms (see in original report of the review)*			
24. or/19–23			

Question components and a selection of relevant terms	Type of terms		Boolean operator
	Free	MeSH	(*see glossary*)
18 and 24			AND (combines *population* and *intervention* and *study designs*)
25. limit 25 to human			

Commands and symbols for Ovid MEDLINE

$ Truncation, e.g. antibiotic$ will pick up antibiotics in general as well as different types of antibiotics (e.g. antibiotics, aminoglycosides; antibiotics, lactam)

adj   Proximity and adjacency searching, e.g. chronic adj wounds$ means that these terms appear next to each other

.tw   Textword search, e.g. skin adj ulcer.tw will search for these adjacent textwords in title or abstract

/   Medical subject heading (MeSH) search, e.g. diabetic foot/ will search for MeSH in indexing terms

The original search is part of the full report of the review available at www.ncchta.org/ execsumm/summ421.htm.

comparability of groups at baseline for severity of ulcers was particularly important because there were concerns about inadequacies of methods used for minimizing selection bias. Assessment of the wound healing process to determine *outcomes* is critical even when measurement bias is minimized by blinding *outcome* assessors. This is because *outcome* assessment could be qualitatively different. For example, when assessing healing, the *outcomes* could be any one of complete healing, ulcer healing quotient, healing index, improvement scores, etc. Complete healing should be regarded as the most important *outcome* due to its importance to patients. Considering both generic and specific issues, a quality checklist with a total of nine items can be developed as shown in Box C3.3.

This checklist is applied to studies included in the review (Box C3.4), but the quality is often unclear due to lack of reporting. Where information on quality is available, many studies fall short of meeting the desired quality. For example, even when studies purport to be randomized, there are deficiencies both in sequence generation and in allocation concealment.

Step 4: Summarizing the evidence

A brief descriptive summary of the studies' characteristics and effects is tabulated in Box C3.5. A number of treatment comparisons were available but only in studies with a small number of patients (range 8–52 per group). Duration of follow-up also varied (range 2–20 weeks) and there was no consistency in

Box C3.3 A quality assessment checklist for studies on effectiveness of antimicrobials for chronic wounds

The clinical question and selection criteria

- Nature of question   Assessment of effectiveness
- Study design   Evaluation of effectiveness of therapy, focusing on how one treatment compares with another (*see Box 1.4*)
- Study design threshold   Inclusion criteria: Randomized controlled trials (*see Box 5.2*)
                Experimental studies without randomization
                Cohort studies with concurrent controls
           Exclusion criteria: Studies with historical controls
                Case-control studies

The quality checklist

a) Generic quality items for checklist (see also Boxes 3.2 and 3.3)

- **Adequate generation of random sequence for allocating patients to interventions**
  Computer generated random numbers or random numbers tables
- **Adequate concealment of allocation**
  Robust methods to prevent foreknowledge of the allocation sequence to clinicians and patients, e.g. centralized real-time or pharmacy-controlled randomization in unblinded studies, or serially numbered identical containers in blinded studies
- **Adequate blinding**
  Care provider, study patients and outcome assessors
- ***A priori* sample size estimation**
- **Description of withdrawals**
  Numbers and reasons provided for each group
- **Intention-to-treat analysis** (ITT)
  Inclusion of all those who dropped out/were lost to follow-up in the analysis so that the calculations indeed follow the ITT principle

b) Specific quality items related to clinical features of the review question

- **The population**
  Correct inclusion/exclusion criteria
  Comparison of severity of wound condition at baseline
- **The interventions**
  No items
- **The outcome**
  Importance of outcomes: complete healing (critical); ulcer healing quotient, healing index, improvement scores and microbial growth (surrogates))

See Box C3.4 for description of study quality

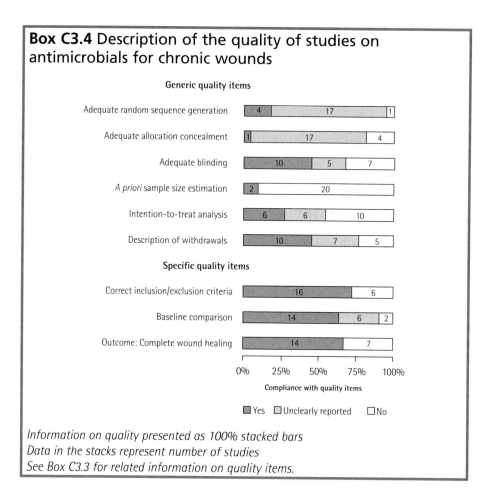

Box C3.4 Description of the quality of studies on antimicrobials for chronic wounds

Generic quality items

Adequate random sequence generation	4 / 17 / 1
Adequate allocation concealment	1 / 17 / 4
Adequate blinding	10 / 5 / 7
A priori sample size estimation	2 / 20
Intention-to-treat analysis	6 / 6 / 10
Description of withdrawals	10 / 7 / 5

Specific quality items

Correct inclusion/exclusion criteria	16 / 6
Baseline comparison	14 / 6 / 2
Outcome: Complete wound healing	14 / 7

0% 25% 50% 75% 100%
Compliance with quality items

■ Yes ☐ Unclearly reported ☐ No

Information on quality presented as 100% stacked bars
Data in the stacks represent number of studies
See Box C3.3 for related information on quality items.

measures of *outcomes*. This variation in what is done to whom, over what period and how *outcomes* are assessed, introduces clinical heterogeneity and this makes a meaningful synthesis of results difficult (and makes meta-analysis impossible).

An examination of the observed effects in individual studies shows large values for point estimates of odds ratios (OR), but most effects are not statistically significant as the 95% confidence intervals (CI) include the possibility of no beneficial effect or even a harmful effect. For example, Wunderlich (1991) found that a silver-based product SIAX was better than various control regimens with an OR of 3.9 but the 95% CI is 0.7–22.1. Similarly,

Heterogeneity is the variation of effects between studies. It may arise because of differences between studies in key characteristics of their *populations*, *interventions* and *outcomes* (clinical heterogeneity), and their *study designs* and quality (methodological heterogeneity).

Effect is a measure of association between an *intervention* and an *outcome*.

Point estimate of effect is its observed value in a study.

Confidence interval is the imprecision in the point estimate, i.e. the range around it within which the 'true' value of the effect can be expected to lie with a given degree of certainty (95%). This reflects uncertainty due to play of chance.

Alinovi (1986) showed that healing rate was worse when standard care was supplemented by systemic antibiotics compared with standard care alone with an OR of 0.54, but 95% CI is 0.1–1.9. Even when effects were statistically significant, e.g. Morias (1979) reports OR 20.3 (95% CI 1.1–375.1), the estimation is quite imprecise due to small sample size. Considering the low quality of the studies, one could hardly be enthused to trust such a result, even when it is statistically significant.

Step 5: Interpreting the findings

This review shows that research on the value of different antimicrobial products in wound care is scarce. Despite an exhaustive search effort, there are only a few relevant studies (Box C3.1) and their quality is relatively low (Box C3.4). A descriptive summary of the evidence shows that the observed effects are seemingly good (perhaps one reason why these studies are published despite their low quality), but they are imprecise, as insufficient numbers of patients are studied (Box C3.5). Technically speaking, the studies are likely to be underpowered. In this situation, the studies are unable to detect an effect when one possibly exists, so one cannot prove the lack of effectiveness of the *interventions*. None of the numerous antimicrobials currently in use for various types of chronic ulcers has been robustly assessed, i.e. with appropriate design and conduct, clinically relevant *outcomes* and large enough sample size. Thus, no recommendations can be made regarding superiority or lack of effectiveness of any of the antimicrobial agents. Needless to say, additional research is needed.

Power is the ability of a study to statistically demonstrate an effect when one exists. It is related to sample size. The larger the sample size, the more the power, and the lower the risk that a possible effect could be missed.

Resolution of the scenario

You are taken by surprise about the slim and feeble body of evidence on such a common problem as chronic wounds, which have a significant impact on healthcare resources in your primary healthcare setting. For you, it is currently not possible to inform a clinical policy on the management of chronic wounds with robust evidence.

Lack of evidence of effectiveness does not equate with evidence of lack of effectiveness! So you decide to form the most sensible policy using common sense and the consensus of your colleagues (this keeps everyone happy). However, you obtain agreement to periodically seek new evidence and update your policy when new robust evidence becomes available.

To help fill the gap in evidence that you have identified through this review, there are some other options open to you. To help generate the new evidence:

- the least you can do is submit this topic to relevant research funding bodies for prioritization

Box C3.5 A brief summary of the findings of studies included in a systematic review on antimicrobials for chronic wounds

(not all comparisons included in the original review are presented in this table)

Population subgroups	Interventions (number of patients/ulcers in group)		Outcomes		Effects
Study author & year of publication	Control group (standard/placebo)	Experimental group	Observation period	Outcome measure[+]	Effect estimate* (95% CI)
Diabetic ulcer					
Systemic treatments					
Chanteleau 1996	Placebo (22)	Antibiotics (22)	3 weeks	Complete healing	OR: 0.45 (0.1–1.6)
Lipsky 1990	Cephalexin (29)	Clindamycin (27)	2 weeks	Complete healing	OR: 1.31 (0.4–4.0)
Topical treatments					
Vandeputte (unpublished)	Hydrogel (15)	Chlorhexidine (14)	12 weeks	Complete healing	OR: 0.07 (0.007–0.7)
Venous ulcer					
Systemic treatments					
Huovinen 1994	Ciprofloxacin (12)	Trimethoprim (12)	12 weeks	Complete healing	OR: 2.14 (0.38–12.2)
Alinovi 1986	Standard (24)	Antibiotics+ standard (24)	3 weeks	Complete healing	OR: 0.54 (0.1–1.9)
Topical treatments					
Pierard-Franchimont 1997	Hydrocolloid (21)	Povidone iodine + hydrocolloid (21)	8 weeks	Median healing index	ES: 1.00 (−0.4–2.4)
Bishop 1992	Placebo (29)	Silver sulphadiazine (30)	4 weeks	Complete healing	OR: 7.57 (0.8–67.4)
Cameron 1991	Non-medicated tulle gras (15)	Mupirocin-impregnated tulle gras (15)	12 weeks	Complete healing	OR: 1.31 (0.31–5.49)
Salim 1991	Allopurinol (51)	Dimethyl sulphoxide (50)	12 weeks	Complete healing	OR: 2.04 (0.36–11.69)
Wunderlich 1991	Various preparations (20)	Silver impregnated activated charcoal dressing (20)	6 weeks	Complete healing	OR: 3.86 (0.7–22.1)
Blair 1988	Saline (30)	Silver sulphadiazine (30)	12 weeks	Complete healing	OR: 0.43 (0.14–1.38)

Study	Control	Experimental	Until healed	Outcome	Effect estimate
Pegum 1968	Lint (17)	Polynaxylin + lint (17)	Until healed	Mean ulcer healing quotient	ES: -0.30 mm²/day (-2.1-1.5)
Pressure ulcers					
Topical treatments					
Della Marchina 1997	Alternative spray (10)	Antiseptic spray (9)	15 days	Complete healing	OR: 2.57 (0.19-34.6)
Toba 1997	Povidone iodine/sugar (11)	Gentian violet 0.1% blended with dibutyryl cAMP (8)	14 weeks	Mean % baseline ulcer area remaining	ES: 11.1 (-8.69-30.89)
Gerding 1992	AtD ointment (13)	DermaMend (26)	4 weeks	No. of improved scores	OR: 6.57 (1.30-33.34)
Huchon 1992	Hydrocolloid (38)	Povidone iodine (38)	8 weeks	Improved scores	OR: 0.46 (0.2-1.4)
Chronic ulcers of mixed aetiology					
Systemic treatments					
Valtonen 1989	Disinfectant (8)	Ciprofloxacin + disinfectant (18)	12 weeks	Complete healing	OR: 3.84 (0.2-83.5)
Morias 1979	Placebo (29)	Levamisole (30)	20 weeks	Complete healing	OR: 20.33 (1.1-375.1)
Topical treatments					
Worsley 1991	Hydrocolloid (12)	Povidone iodine ointment (15)	12 weeks	Complete healing	OR: 0.31 (0.05-2.08)
Beitner 1985	Saline (10)	Benzoyl peroxide 20% (10)	6 weeks	Mean % remaining ulcer area	ES: 34.10 (21.1-47.1)
Margraf 1977	Various agents (10)	Silver zinc allantoine cream (10)	Until healed	Mean days to heal	ES 59.0 (34.12-83.88)
Marzin 1982	Benzoyl peroxide (20)	Collagen gel (20)	12 weeks	Wound area remaining	No effect estimate reported (p < 0.01)

+ In studies with several outcome measures the most clinically important one is presented using the following hierarchy: complete healing > ulcer healing quotient, healing index, improvement scores > microbial growth.

* Odds ratio (OR) >1 and effect size (ES) > 0 indicates improved outcome with experimental treatment. See Box 4.1 for advice on constructing tables.

- you can also design and commence a robust clinical trial yourself if you are so inclined and can obtain the funding to do this
- the most practical approach in our view is to actively recruit patients in a relevant clinical trial if there is one ongoing.

An update of the review in this case study showed that there have been four additional studies. The methodological quality of all studies was only moderate due to unclear concealment of the treatment allocation, unclear or lack of blinding and their uncertain use of intention-to-treat analysis. The studies were generally small, three included 21 or fewer patients in each treatment arm, whereas the fourth study had more than 100 patients per arm. Only one trial reported a clinically relevant outcome (complete healing rate), while the others measured surrogates, e.g. change in ulcer surface area, which may or may not be a valid proxy for complete healing. How could this new information fill the knowledge gap you identified? There was weak evidence that topical preparations like cadexomer iodine improved ulcer healing compared to standard care. No evidence supported the routine use of systemic antibiotics. You could inform your colleagues about the review, and may decide to modify the care protocol for patients with chronic wounds, with a weak recommendation favouring the use of cadexomer iodine.

● Case study 4:
Reviewing evidence on accuracy of a test

Step 1
Framing questions
↓
Step 2
Identifying relevant
literature
↓
Step 3
Assessing quality of
the literature
↓
Step 4
Summarizing the
evidence
↓
Step 5
Interpreting the
findings

No document of approximately 1800 words can purport to do justice to systematic reviews of test accuracy literature. We make no attempt to profess mastery of the methodological nuances in this expanding and, for some, exciting field.

In this case study, we reinforce the general principles behind systematic reviews by demonstrating their application in a scenario concerning use of evidence about accuracy of a test. It provides a good demonstration of study quality assessment, exploration of heterogeneity, quantitative synthesis and interpretation of findings.

Scenario: Ultrasound scan test for postmenopausal women with vaginal bleeding

You are a clinician responsible for women's health in a primary care centre serving a relatively large retired *population*. You are often faced with women who present with unexpected episodes of vaginal bleeding after menopause. You know that in the past these patients used to be routinely investigated by gynaecologists using uterine curettage under anaesthesia. This practice is now considered outdated, but current local practice still involves referral to a specialist based in a tertiary care setting. You wonder if an ultrasound scan of the uterus can exclude pathology accurately in postmenopausal women with abnormal vaginal bleeding. In this way, women who test negative will not need referral to tertiary care.

You search MEDLINE using PubMed Clinical Queries to see if there are any reviews in the literature. At www.ncbi.nlm. nih.gov/entrez/query/static/clinical.html you type 'ultrasound postmenopausal bleeding' in the query box of the Systematic Reviews feature and click the Go button. You find the following seemingly relevant citations on this topic:

- Evaluation of the woman with postmenopausal bleeding: Society of Radiologists in Ultrasound-Sponsored Consensus Conference statement. *J Ultrasound Med* 2001; **20**: 1025–36. (this is not a review)
- Ultrasonographic endometrial thickness for diagnosing endometrial pathology in women with postmenopausal bleeding: a meta-analysis. *Acta Obstet Gynecol Scand* 2002; **81**: 799–816.

This case study was developed as a learning aid in 2002. An update search carried out for the second edition of this book revealed no further review that was incompatible with the conclusions of the original case study. So we decided to keep this case study in the same form as it was presented in the first edition.

Step 1: Framing the question

Free form question

Among postmenopausal women with abnormal vaginal bleeding, does ultrasound scan exclude uterine cancer accurately?

Structured question

The population	Postmenopausal women in the community with symptoms of vaginal bleeding.
The test	Endometrial thickness measurement during ultrasound imaging of the pelvis and the uterus (see Box C4.1). You are mainly interested in the accuracy of the negative test result.
The reference standard	Endometrial cancer confirmed histologically. There are many abnormalities of the endometrium and the uterus (benign, pre-cancer and cancer). Among your *population*, endometrial cancer is the most important one. Focusing on this diagnosis is not unreasonable (not least for the sake of simplicity in this case). You are mainly interested in excluding the diagnosis of cancer.
The study design	Test accuracy study (Box C4.3), i.e. observational studies in which results of a test (endometrial ultrasound) are compared with the results of a reference standard (endometrial histology).

Step 2: Identifying relevant literature

An electronic search was carried out to capture all the relevant citations about ultrasound of the endometrium and then those citations identified that evaluate ultrasound among postmenopausal women with vaginal bleeding to predict the likelihood of endometrial cancer. MEDLINE and EMBASE databases

Free form question: It describes the query for which you seek an answer through a review in simple language (however vague).

Structured question: Reviewers convert free form questions into a clear and explicit format using a structured approach (see Box 1.2). This makes the query potentially answerable through existing relevant studies.

Question components

The population: A clinically suitable sample of patients

The test: The test whose predictive value is being assessed

The reference standard: A 'gold' standard test that confirms or refutes the diagnosis

The study design: Ways of conducting research to assess the predictive value of the test

Box C4.1 Ultrasound scan of the pelvis and the uterus

In ultrasound imaging of the uterus, the endometrium (lining of the womb) is described in terms of thickness and regularity. Regular endometrium of less than 5 mm thickness is often used to define a threshold or cut-off for abnormality. An example of a normal test result is shown below.

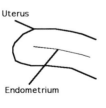
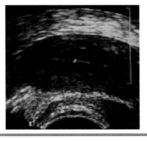

were searched without language restrictions. The search term combination included MeSH, textwords and appropriate word variants of '"ultrasound OR sonography" AND "endometrium OR uterus"'. The resultant set of citations was limited to human studies. The electronic search was coupled with manual scanning of bibliographies of known primary and review articles to identify relevant papers (Box C4.2). In total 57 studies (including 9031 patients) were included in the review. Of these, 21 studies were on the accuracy of endometrial thickness, at a 5 mm abnormality threshold, to predict the diagnosis of endometrial cancer.

Step 3: Assessing study quality

Quality assessment of test accuracy studies

An accuracy study is different from an effectiveness study. It is designed to generate a comparison between measurements obtained by a test and those obtained by a reference standard. A reference standard is a test that confirms or refutes the presence or absence of disease beyond reasonable doubt. Therefore it is sometimes also known as the 'gold' standard. We shall give a basic explanation about the *design* and quality features of a test accuracy study (Box C4.3).

There are many possible sources of bias in accuracy studies, as shown in Box C4.3. Selection bias may arise if the sample is not suitably representative of the *population*. This is less likely to occur when using consecutive or random sampling. Poor descriptions of *test* and *reference standards* in terms of preparation of the patients, details of measurements, computation of results and thresholds for defining abnormality are also associated with bias. The *reference standard* should be a recognized 'gold' standard and it should be administered independently of the *test*. In

Identifying relevant literature
- Develop search term combinations
- Search relevant electronic databases
- Search other relevant resources
- Obtain full papers of potentially relevant citations
- Include/exclude studies using pre-set selection criteria

The **quality** of a study depends on the degree to which its design, conduct and analysis minimizes **biases**.

Bias either exaggerates or underestimates the 'true' accuracy of a *test*.

Box C4.2 Identification of relevant literature on endometrial ultrasound

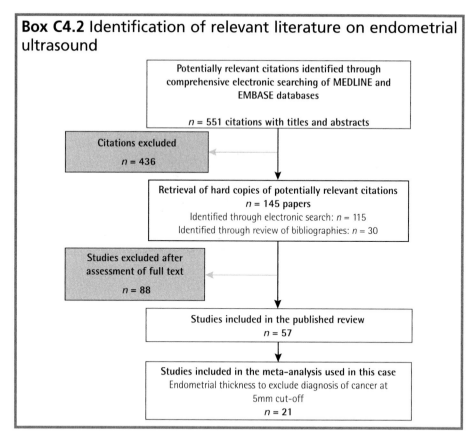

Potentially relevant citations identified through comprehensive electronic searching of MEDLINE and EMBASE databases

n = 551 citations with titles and abstracts

Citations excluded
n = 436

Retrieval of hard copies of potentially relevant citations
n = 145 papers
Identified through electronic search: *n* = 115
Identified through review of bibliographies: *n* = 30

Studies excluded after assessment of full text
n = 88

Studies included in the published review
n = 57

Studies included in the meta-analysis used in this case
Endometrial thickness to exclude diagnosis of cancer at 5mm cut-off
n = 21

addition, observers assessing *reference standards* for verification of diagnosis should be kept blind to measurements obtained from the *test*, and *vice versa*. Blinding avoids bias because recordings made by one observer are not influenced by the knowledge of the measurements obtained by other observers. During the verification process, bias may arise if the *reference standard* is not applied to all patients, or if it is differentially applied to test-positive and test-negative cases.

A detailed quality checklist is developed for assessment of test accuracy studies on endometrial ultrasound using the principles outlined in Step 3. We consider the elements of *study design* (generic items) and couple them with issues relevant to the review question (specific items), as shown in Box C4.3. An overview of the relevant generic aspects of test accuracy studies in this review reveals that the ultrasound *test* and the histological examination of the endometrium, which serves as the *reference standard*, are independent. So the remaining methodological issues related to recruitment of patients, blinding of observers and completeness of verification of diagnosis are examined.

Among quality issues related specifically to the review question, a sufficient description of the *population* to demonstrate that the sample is representative of the disease spectrum seen in practice

Box C4.3 Design and quality of test accuracy studies evaluating endometrial ultrasound

Simple description of study design

An observational study that tests subjects from a relevant population and compares its results with those of a reference standard. For example, studies comparing results of endometrial ultrasound with those of endometrial histology in women with postmenopausal bleeding.

Study flow chart with key generic quality features

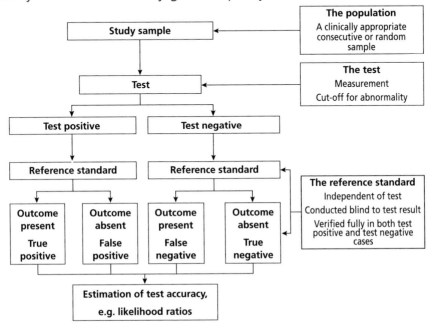

Development of a quality checklist

a) Generic items obtained from the published research appraisal guidelines on test accuracy

- recruitment of subjects (consecutive or random sample)
- independence between the test and the reference standard
- blinding of the observers conducting the reference standard to the findings of the test and vice versa
- verification of diagnosis by reference standard in all tested cases.

b) Specific items related to features of this review

- **The population** Appropriate spectrum composition
- **The test** Adequate description of endometrial ultrasound measurements determining cut-off level for abnormality *a priori*
- **The reference standard** Adequate endometrial samples obtained for reference standard histology. Hysterectomy and directed biopsy are adequate but blind (non-directed) biopsy may be less satisfactory.

See Box C4.4 for results of quality assessment.

is essential, otherwise the estimates of accuracy may be biased. For the *test, a priori* setting of the 5 mm threshold is crucial, as post hoc determination of threshold is subject to manipulation in light of findings of the study. Finally, for the *reference standard*, use of adequate endometrial sampling is crucial to the validity of the selected studies. Adequate methods of obtaining endometrial samples include hysterectomy and directed biopsy.

Study design threshold for study selection

In this review a quality threshold in study selection was used to exclude all studies with case-control design. These studies would have selected cases with and without cancer and patients would be retrospectively examined if their endometrial ultrasound scans were abnormal. Such a design has been empirically shown to be associated with bias, leading to exaggeration of test accuracy.

Description of study quality for selected studies

Box C4.4 indicates the quality of selected studies. For most of the quality items, lack of compliance with good quality features was due to lack of reporting. In general, there were deficiencies of one sort or another among all studies. The impact of these deficiencies on the estimation of accuracy is explored in Box C4.6.

Step 4: Summarizing the evidence

This case study describes the estimates of accuracy of individual studies, the examination of heterogeneity of accuracy across studies and the meta-analysis of individual accuracy estimates among studies using 5-mm thickness as the threshold for abnormality (other details of included studies can be obtained from the original report). But first we must understand how to choose a measure of accuracy (Box C4.5). The discussion about the pros and cons of various accuracy measures is a never-ending story in which there is no consensus among experts and it is outside the remit of this book. To cut a long story short, sensitivity and specificity are often considered to be of a limited clinical value. For the question posed in this case study, you are interested to discover the value of a negative endometrial ultrasound test (at a threshold of 5-mm thickness) for excluding endometrial cancer. This case study describes the statistical synthesis using individual likelihood ratios (LR) for negative test result. For meta-analysis it uses a bivariate model to derive summary LRs. This approach provides the most robust summary estimates, although description of its detail is outside the scope of this book.

Likelihood ratio (LR) is the ratio of the probability of a positive (or negative) test result in subjects with a disease to the probability of the same test result in subjects without the disease. The LR indicates by how much a given test result will raise or lower the probability of having the disease.

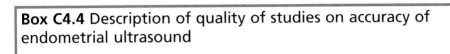

Box C4.4 Description of quality of studies on accuracy of endometrial ultrasound

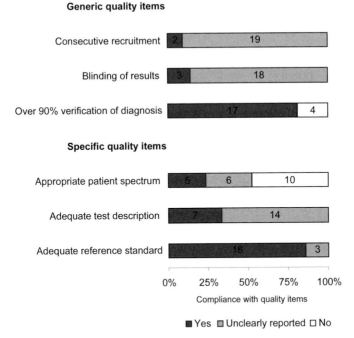

Generic quality items

Consecutive recruitment: 2 | 19

Blinding of results: 3 | 18

Over 90% verification of diagnosis: 17 | 4

Specific quality items

Appropriate patient spectrum: 5 | 6 | 10

Adequate test description: 7 | 14

Adequate reference standard: 18 | 3

0%   25%   50%   75%   100%

Compliance with quality items

■ Yes ▨ Unclearly reported □ No

Information on quality presented as 100% stacked bars
Data in the stacks represent the number of studies
See Box C4.3 for related information on the development of the quality checklist
See Box C4.6 for subgroup analysis.

Variation in test accuracy from study to study

The point estimate of accuracy in each study, its precision (confidence interval) and the possibility of heterogeneity can be explored by examining variability of individual LRs in a Forest plot. As shown in Box C4.6, there is a suspicion about heterogeneity, as confidence intervals do not overlap among some studies. Heterogeneity was confirmed by a formal statistical test. When heterogeneity was found, its possible sources were searched for using subgroup analysis examining the impact of study quality and characteristics (not shown here). No explanation for heterogeneity could be found.

Heterogeneity is the variation of accuracy between studies. It may arise because of differences between studies in key characteristics of their populations, tests and reference standards (clinical heterogeneity), and their study designs and quality (methodological heterogeneity).

Quantitative synthesis of results

In this instance heterogeneity remains unexplained despite an exhaustive exploration. Now do we, or do we not, perform meta-analysis? As discussed in Step 4, caution is required. In this review, authors chose to pool individual LRs using the random effects

Box C4.5 Estimation of accuracy in studies evaluating tests

Measures of test accuracy

These are statistics for summarizing the accuracy of a test. For binary tests, there are three commonly used pairs of accuracy measures: positive and negative predictive values; sensitivity and specificity; and likelihood ratios. Unlike measures of effect, single measures of accuracy are infrequently used.

Computing accuracy for binary test results

A way of computing accuracy measures is shown below. Predictive values give the probability of having a disease and not having a disease among subjects with positive and negative test results respectively. Sensitivity and specificity give the probability of a positive and a negative test result among subjects with and without disease respectively. Likelihood ratios (LRs) describe the relative probabilities of obtaining a test result in subjects with and without a disease. However, with several studies to compute accuracy for and to estimate uncertainty of the accuracy (its confidence intervals), manual calculations can become tedious. We would suggest you use statistical software.

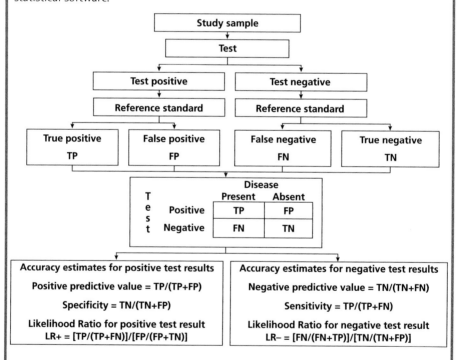

Choosing accuracy measures for binary tests

There is a debate about which measures are preferable and how best to pool them across several studies in a meta-analysis. No single approach is entirely satisfactory. Likelihood ratios (LRs) are more clinically meaningful because when they are used in conjunction with information on disease prevalence (pre-test probability), they help to generate post-test probabilities as shown in Box C4.7. Pooling of individual sensitivity (Sn) and specificity (Sp) results should take into account their interrelationship, as they may not behave independently. Bivariate method and summary receiver operating characteristics plot allows for pooling of results from individual studies taking account of the relation between Sn and Sp. LRs are not suitable for pooling in meta-analysis, particularly when the threshold for abnormality varies from study to study. The preference for LRs over other accuracy measures for clinical interpretation can be met by deriving these from Sn and Sp as LR+ = [Sn/(100–Sp)] and LR– = [(100–Sn0/Sp].

See relevant sections of the glossary for definitions of measures and methods of meta-analysis.

model (not shown in the case study). Precaution was taken to ensure that the summary point estimate was not biased by the choice of this method compared to a fixed effect model. Box C4.6 shows accuracy of the 21 studies evaluating the accuracy of endometrial ultrasound using LR–, sensitivity and specificity. A meta-analysis using a bivariate model produced summary sensitivity and specificity from which LRs were derived: LR– was 0.025 (95% CI 0.005–0.118). Interestingly the summary LR+ for positive test is 2.14 (95% CI 1.75–2.61) although this information was not really required to help with decision making in your case scenario.

Bivariate model estimates the correlation between sensitivity and specificity and incorporates this in meta-analysis of results from test accuracy studies.

Box C4.6 Exploring reasons for variation in accuracy among studies evaluating endometrial ultrasound

Forest plot

Summary of likelihood ratios for negative test results (LR–) among studies with an endometrial ultrasound test threshold of 5 mm thickness (sorted in alphabetical order).

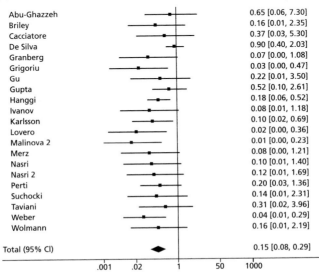

Abu-Ghazzeh	0.65 [0.06, 7.30]
Briley	0.16 [0.01, 2.35]
Cacciatore	0.37 [0.03, 5.30]
De Silva	0.90 [0.40, 2.03]
Granberg	0.07 [0.00, 1.08]
Grigoriu	0.03 [0.00, 0.47]
Gu	0.22 [0.01, 3.50]
Gupta	0.52 [0.10, 2.61]
Hanggi	0.18 [0.06, 0.52]
Ivanov	0.08 [0.01, 1.18]
Karlsson	0.10 [0.02, 0.69]
Lovero	0.02 [0.00, 0.36]
Malinova 2	0.01 [0.00, 0.23]
Merz	0.08 [0.00, 1.21]
Nasri	0.10 [0.01, 1.40]
Nasri 2	0.12 [0.01, 1.69]
Perti	0.20 [0.03, 1.36]
Suchocki	0.14 [0.01, 2.31]
Taviani	0.31 [0.02, 3.96]
Weber	0.04 [0.01, 0.29]
Wolmann	0.16 [0.01, 2.19]
Total (95% CI)	0.15 [0.08, 0.29]

.001 .02 1 50 1000

Plot of sensitivity *vs* specificity

Sensitivities and specificities among studies with an endometrial ultrasound test threshold of 5 mm thickness are shown with empty circles. Summary estimate of sensitivity (98%; 95% CI 93-99%) and specificity (53%; 95% CI 44–63%) obtained using bivariate model is shown with a filled square and its confidence intervals shown with a dotted ellipse around the square. Likelihood ratios can be derived from these estimates as LR+ = [Sn/(100–Sp)] and LR− = [(100–Sn0/Sp].

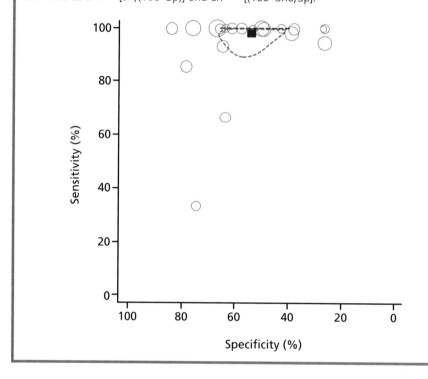

Step 5: Interpreting the findings

The prevalence of endometrial cancer varies according to age. So the likelihood or probability of cancer given a negative ultrasound test result will also vary. The changes in probability produced by the summary LR− can be mathematically computed or they can be estimated using a nomogram (see Box C4.7). A negative test result virtually eliminates the possibility of endometrial cancer among younger women; however, it may not substantially reduce the probability among older women (in our view).

Resolution of scenario

The answer to your question 'does a pelvic ultrasound scan exclude uterine cancer accurately in postmenopausal women with abnormal vaginal bleeding?' has to be 'yes, for many of your patients'. A negative result at less than 5 mm endometrial

Pre-test probability is an estimate of probability of disease before tests are carried out. It is usually based on disease prevalence.

Post-test probability is an estimate of probability of disease in light of information obtained from testing. With accurate tests, the post-test estimates of probabilities change substantially from pre-test estimates.

Box C4.7 The impact of a negative test result in endometrial ultrasound (at a 5-mm threshold) on the likelihood of endometrial cancer among postmenopausal women with vaginal bleeding

Generating post-test probabilities

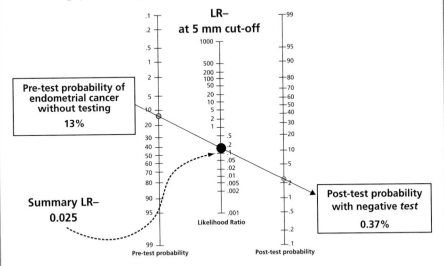

Nomogram adapted from *N Engl J Med* 1975; **293**: 257.
See Box C4.6 for summary likelihood ratio for negative text result, LR–

Post-test probabilities of endometrial cancer according to risk groups based on age

Age group	Pre-test probability*	Post-test probability+
<50 years	0.5%	0.01%
51-60 years	1.0%	0.03%
>60 years	13.0%	0.37%

* *Obtained from population based data*

+ Computed using the following formula:

$$\text{Post-test probability} = \frac{\text{Likelihood ratio} \times \text{Pre-test probability}}{[1 - \text{Pre-test probability} \times (1 - \text{Likelihood ratio})]}$$

thickness rules out endometrial cancer with good certainty among low risk patients (e.g. age < 60 years), so there should be no need for you to refer them to tertiary care. It is important to remember that there is always a chance of a false-negative test result, even among low risk patients. So, if patients remain symptomatic, they will need further evaluation. For high risk patients (e.g. age > 60 years) you don't have good certainty in ruling out disease from a negative ultrasound test, so you might even refer them on to tertiary care without ultrasound testing. Needless to say, your low risk patients with ultrasound endometrial thickness greater than 5 mm would need to be investigated further to ascertain presence or absence of pathology in a tertiary care setting.

● Case study 5:
Reviewing qualitative evidence to evaluate patient experience

Elaine Denny

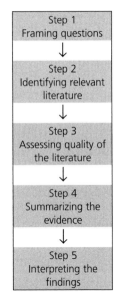

Step 1
Framing questions
↓
Step 2
Identifying relevant literature
↓
Step 3
Assessing quality of the literature
↓
Step 4
Summarizing the evidence
↓
Step 5
Interpreting the findings

The purpose of qualitative research is to explore experience and to seek understanding and explanation. Through quantitative research one may discover that an intervention is effective, but will patients find it acceptable? Will carers provide it? What will facilitate its implementation? What will hinder it? Answers to these and other related questions lie in exploration of subjective experiences of people. There has been an increasing recognition within health that many issues such as acceptability of interventions cannot fully be captured by quantitative means. Clinicians and practitioners need to allow people to relate their experience and the way in which they interpret their world in order to understand their concerns better. Researchers need to study these subjective phenomena to help improve the insight practitioners and policy makers have. Thus there has been an increasing amount of health-related qualitative research and an interest in summarizing findings of qualitative papers in a rigorous way using the tools of systematic review, aiding evidence-based practice.

Primary qualitative research deals with very individual responses of study participants. This approach does not generate statistical averages and it can sometimes be erroneously assumed that this leads to problems in conducting systematic reviews. The reality is not so bleak. Systematic reviews can be used to integrate research findings in a structured way regardless of whether the primary studies are quantitative or qualitative. The results generated by individual qualitative studies can be collated and synthesized to gain new insights. Qualitative reviewers do this through metasynthesis, a technique that seeks to gain further understanding and explanations of the phenomena researched in primary studies.

This case study will demonstrate how to employ reviews of qualitative research to enrich evidence-based medicine. It will demonstrate how the key points about appraisal shown at the end of each Step in this book can be employed to evaluate such reviews for their trustworthiness and usefulness.

Qualitative research seeks to understand the way people make sense of events and experience.

Quantitative research involves the collection of data in numerical form, or that which can be converted to numeric form for analysis.

Metasynthesis: The synthesis of existing qualitative research findings on a specific research question. This does not involve meta-analysis.

Scenario: The experience of endometriosis

You are a general practitioner in a busy practice, and you have just had a long consultation with a young woman. She presented with chronic pelvic pain and also found sexual intercourse very painful, which was affecting her relationship with her partner. She told you that the pain was constantly there, although it was worse around menstruation, and that she was at the end of her tether. You knew from her records that over the years she had consulted with some of your colleagues who had prescribed non-steroidal anti-inflammatory analgesia and oral contraception, but nothing so far had relieved the pain. Your colleagues had suspected that she was exaggerating the pain associated with normal menstruation. When you questioned how long this had been going on she replied that it had been ten years. Having browsed the Internet, she suspected that her symptoms may be caused by endometriosis. You referred her to a gynaecologist, who carried out a laparoscopy. This confirmed the diagnosis of endometriosis. You wondered whether referral could have been made earlier.

A MEDLINE search using the search term 'endometriosis' revealed a plethora of basic science and clinical papers, many of the latter commenting on the delay in diagnosing endometriosis and the poor experience of women within the health system. In order to feel better equipped to manage similar patients in the future, you decided to find out whether this woman's experience was typical of endometriosis. Qualitative research findings will elaborate on the experience of women with endometriosis.

This case study will utilize the paper:

- Systematic reviews of qualitative evidence: What are the experiences of women with endometriosis? *J Obstet Gynaecol* 2006: **26**: 501-6.

Step 1: Framing the question

Free form question

How does the experience of endometriosis impact on women's lives?

Structured question

The population	Women with a confirmed diagnosis of endometriosis.
The interventions	Either observation or treatment for endometriosis.
The outcomes	Effects on pain, work and social relationships, self-image, etc.
The study design	Interviews, focus groups, diary keeping.

Question components

The population: A clinically suitable sample of patients.

The interventions: Comparison of groups with and without the intervention.

The outcomes: Changes in health status, social relationships, self-image, etc due to interventions.

The study design: Ways of conducting research to assess the effects of interventions.

Note that the question does not pose a statistically testable hypothesis as the outcomes are described subjectively by study participants rather than quantified numerically.

Step 2: Identifying relevant studies

A search of MEDLINE using the search term endometriosis revealed 12 546 citations. The majority were reports of quantitative studies. Using filters for qualitative research to narrow the search to qualitative studies produced 192 citations. However, the majority of these papers did not have a qualitative methodology and endometriosis was not the primary focus of the research. From this search, only four papers fulfilled the selection criteria based on the structured question above. The major social science search engines (ASSIA, QUALIDATA, REGARD and the Social Science Citation index) were searched using the following key terms: endometriosis, pain, self-image and terms for qualitative methodology (Box C5.1). From these searches and from reference lists, a further four qualitative studies on living with endometriosis emerged, giving eight peer reviewed studies for this review (Box C5.2).

As in all good reviews, the process concerning study selection and the decisions regarding selection should be transparent. In reviews of qualitative research, this is particularly important when different study designs are to be considered simultaneously (Box C5.3). There is a debate around whether studies using different methods should be combined in a review, although some argue

Identifying relevant literature
- Develop search term combinations
- Search relevant electronic databases
- Search other relevant resources
- Obtain full papers of potentially relevant citations
- Include/exclude studies using pre-set selection criteria

Study design filter employs a search term combination to capture citations of studies with a particular design.

Box C5.1 Some important databases of qualitative research in healthcare

ASSIA

Applied Social Sciences Index and Abstracts is an indexing and abstracting database that covers health, social services, psychology, sociology, economics and politics.

QUALIDATA

ESDS Qualidata is a specialist service of the Economic and Social Data Service (ESDS) that acquires digital data collections from qualitative and mixed methods contemporary research and from UK-based 'classic studies'. Users are able to locate accessible sources of qualitative data across the UK.

ESRC Society Today (formerly REGARD)

This site contains all research funded by the Economic and Social Science Research Council, and summaries and final reports of research projects can be searched.

Social Science Citation Index

This is accessed via the Web of Science and provides citation information that enables researchers to source research data.

Searching for qualitative studies

See Section 2.1.3 for searching for study designs. A qualitative research design filter can be used to restrict the citations of initial searches to those with a qualitative methodology. Due to its in-depth thesaurus terms, CINAHL is generally accepted as a good database to find qualitative research articles. In CINAHL exploding 'qualitative research' will include 'action research', 'ethnographic research', 'grounded theory', 'naturalistic inquiry' and 'phenomenological research'. Other terms that can be part of a qualitative research filter include: interviews.exp (includes structured interview, semi-structured interview, unstructured interview); observational methods. exp (includes non-participant observation, participant observation); focus groups; narratives; diary keeping.

Box C5.2 Identification of relevant literature on experiences of women with endometriosis

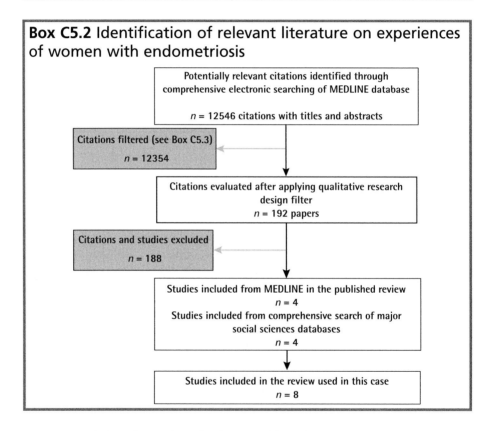

that such restrictions detract from the richness of data obtained. In this review the selection was not restricted by qualitative research method.

Step 3: Assessing study quality

There have been a number of methods developed by which to assess the quality of qualitative studies, although it is not appropriate to have a formulaic approach to determine the quality of this type of research.

Box C5.3 Some important study designs for qualitative research in healthcare

Interviewing Questioning people about their views or experience of a phenomenon or event. Can range from structured, where each participant is asked the same questions, to unstructured, which consists of a list of broad areas to be covered, the exact format of each interview being determined as it progresses.

Focus group The collection of qualitative data using a group interview on a topic chosen by the researcher. Usually 6–12 people are involved, and they can be used to gauge issues of importance to interested parties in order to develop an interview schedule, or as a research method in their own right.

Diary keeping A qualitative research method, usually an addition to questionnaire or interview data, where participants record experience and emotions contemporaneously. Can be free form, where people write what they want to, or structured where they have specific questions to answer or topics to write about.

In this review, the framework for the study of quality assessment paid particular attention to the validity with which studies captured the meaning that women put on their experience. From this an insight or understanding develops of the experience of endometriosis. A set of questions was formulated to be addressed when reading each of the articles in order to assess quality (Box C5.4). These need to be used with sensitivity in order to allow a qualitative critical appraisal. As this is a subjective process, it is crucial that quality assessment is initially undertaken by at least two reviewers acting independently, who then come together to formulate an agreed assessment. One important element of systematic review of qualitative research is the notion of generalization (Box C5.4). Within qualitative research the aim is not to extrapolate to wider populations, but to add to the understanding of a phenomenon. So in this case we would want to know how far the findings of the studies in the review concur with other studies that provide insight into the experience of endometriosis.

> The **quality** of a qualitative research study depends on the degree to which its design, conduct and analysis is trustworthy. Trustworthiness consists of several concepts including credibility, dependability, transferability, confirmability.

Step 4: Summarizing the evidence

The reporting of narrative is a common method of presentation of findings in primary qualitative studies. In a systematic review these can be collated and synthesized. This is usually accomplished by the generation of themes, which can initially be done by using the key areas identified within each selected study which is carried out by reviewing published findings, rather than re-analysing original data. Reading and re-reading the studies will result in the

Box C5.4 Description of quality of studies on experiences of women with endometriosis

Key issues on which the quality of qualitative research studies is judged

- Qualitative research gives a voice to participants, which allows them to talk about their experience; therefore research findings should reflect their perspective and not that of the researcher.
- Qualitative research design should be flexible enough for adaptation as perspectives of participants are revealed, but without losing rigour.
- The sample should be purposive, that is drawn from the population that has the experience. However, it should not be so narrowly drawn that only certain experiences get reported. For example, sampling from self-help groups will often attract participants with negative experiences.
- Transparency in each stage of the research process is vital in a flexible and responsive research design.
- Different sources of knowledge are usually consulted for the literature review, and the extent to which the study under review conforms to or refutes this can be gauged.
- How the research moves through these stages should be explicit and justified. Often this will be an iterative process, in which case an explanation as to how each stage is influenced by the previous one should be given.
- Qualitative research is context specific and so the aim is to increase understanding. There should be a discussion of the extent to which the findings are consistent with those from similar studies.

Description of study quality

Information on quality is presented as 100% stacked bars. Data in the stacks represent the number of studies.

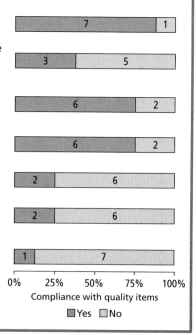

Does the research as reported illuminate the subjective meaning and context of those being researched?

Is there evidence of adaption and responsiveness of the research design to the circumstances and issues of real life social settings met during the study course?

Does the sample produce the type of knowledge necessary to understand the structures and processes within which the individuals or situations are located?

Is the description provided detailed enough to allow the reader to interpret the context and meaning of what is being researched?

Are different sources of knowledge about the same issue compared and contrasted?

Does the research move from description of the data, through quotation or examples, to an analysis and interpretation of the meaning and significance?

Are claims being made for the consistency of the findings to either other bodies of knowledge or to other populations or groups?

Compliance with quality items

■ Yes □ No

development and possible merging of further themes. This process can be facilitated by the use of qualitative data handling software (Box C5.5).

The themes formulated in this way allow synthesis of the qualitative findings. This integration of studies is analogous to the pooling of data in a quantitative review. It is important that during this process the original meaning of the work is not lost. Similarities in the studies can be identified and categorized using the identified or emergent themes. Aberrant findings can be explored to elicit an explanation. In this way a reviewer gets a picture of the phenomenon under study, in this case the experience of living with endometriosis.

> **Phenomenon** is an occurrence or a fact. It is often used as a generic term for the object of a research study.

The reliability of summarizing qualitative evidence and interpretation of findings (Steps 4 and 5) can be improved in one of two ways. Where there is a research team, each member conducts steps 4 and 5 independently. They will then agree emerging themes and iron out inconsistencies, which need to be made transparent in subsequent reports or publications. Alternatively Steps 4 and 5 can be independently verified by someone outside of the team who has expertise in the research issue.

In the endometriosis studies reviewed, detailed narrative was reported but analysis of the data was limited. Common themes were identified from the articles, but no article reported on all of these themes apart from pain. Nevertheless, similar results were reported by all studies. As pain was the one common theme, it provides a useful example of how findings can be synthesized. Various descriptions of pain were given in the articles. In three of these articles individual narrative from participants in the research was reported in the words of the author(s) as representative

> **Theme** is an idea that is developed by the coding of qualitative data. The large quantities of data produced by a qualitative study are managed by the generation of themes and the coding of parts of the data to each theme. The perspectives of each research participant on each theme can be compared and analysed.

Box C5.5 A simple overview of qualitative data synthesis

- Data collected in qualitative research can include transcripts of interviews, group discussions, observation, reflective field notes, etc.
- The analysis of qualitative data involves interpretation of these transcripts to form impressions. Coding is an interpretive technique that requires the researcher to read the text and demarcate segments within it. Each segment is labelled with a word or short phrase that suggests how the associated data segments inform the research objectives. When coding is complete, the researcher can discuss similarities and differences in codes across transcripts. This forms the basis for organizing and reporting results.
- The use of qualitative data handling software can assist in analysis of large quantities of data, by categorizing it according to codes generated by the researcher. This way data on a particular phenomenon can be retrieved quickly from every transcript.
- Using the example of endometriosis pain, all references to pain in the interview transcripts may be entered into the software under the code of 'pain'. Sub codes of 'pelvic pain', 'dyspareunia', etc may also be used to categorize the data. The researcher can later retrieve all references to pain from the entire participant group at the click of a mouse.

of the group as a whole. The remaining papers gave examples of descriptions of pain from individual women, with terms such as 'intense', 'a knife going into each ovary', 'stabbing' and 'tremendous' being frequently used. This is unlikely to be captured by the linear pain scales of quantitative research.

In synthesizing this information we can conclude that pain was a constant theme in all qualitative research on endometriosis. In three studies this was described by the authors from unreported data, but five studies reported women's own descriptions of the quality and severity of pain. Seven of the studies also reported how the experience of pain impacted on quality of life, e.g. on work and social relationships. In four of the studies women described how their social life had suffered, with friends and family losing patience when planned events were continually cancelled. Relationships with partners were also negatively affected, although one study did point to partners as offering the major support to women with endometriosis. Three studies found that women who took time off work due to pain felt guilty, and were often disbelieved by colleagues and employers, sometimes being made to feel they were malingering.

Step 5: Interpreting the findings

This case scenario focused on the experience of endometriosis reported in a systematic review of qualitative research. It revealed that the experience of endometriosis has a profound negative effect on the lives of women. Despite a comprehensive search of relevant databases, only a few studies of variable quality were found. They provided detailed narrative but analyses were limited. As one purpose of qualitative research is the generation of new theory to explain a phenomenon, this lack of analysis is a limitation of the reviewed research.

Theory is abstract knowledge or reasoning as a way of explaining social relations. Theory may influence research (deduction), or research may lead to the development of theory (induction).

Resolution of scenario

By conducting this systematic review and evaluating the studies you have gained a better understanding of your own patient's experience, and have discovered that her history is a familiar one. You could not have gained this insight by reading clinical papers that focus on the effectiveness of different treatments rather than on the impact of living with endometriosis. The research that was retrieved tended to report and analyse women's comments, but did not do so from any particular theoretical perspective (e.g. psychology). However, your understanding of women's experience has improved and this may influence your management of similar patients in the future.

Since this review was undertaken more qualitative papers on endometriosis have been published, substantiating the main findings of this review.

● Case study 6:
Reviewing evidence on the effects of educational interventions

Sharon Buckley

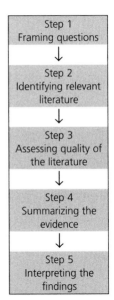

Medical educationalists increasingly use systematic reviews to evaluate the effects of educational interventions. Peculiarities of electronic databases and inherent complexities of primary educational research make systematic reviews in this field challenging. However, such reviews can provide valuable insights into the available evidence about particular effects of teaching methods on student learning, guiding resource allocation and supporting educational practice.

This case study will explore the specific issues relating to systematic reviews of the effects of educational interventions. Based on a published review, it will consider the requirements for literature searching and quality assessment in the educational context. It will demonstrate an approach to synthesis of educational research evidence when meta-analysis is not appropriate.

Scenario: effects of portfolios on student learning in undergraduate medical education

You are an Education Development Specialist based in a large medical and nursing school. Your faculty is considering introducing a professional development portfolio for all its undergraduate medical students. Views on whether, how and when the portfolio should be introduced are mixed: some faculty view portfolios as an ideal preparation for postgraduate medical education and lifelong learning, others as a drain on scarce resources that emphasizes reflection at the expense of essential clinical knowledge and understanding. You are keen that any decisions about curriculum development should be based on the best available evidence as to the effects of using a portfolio on undergraduate student learning. You have identified the following Best Evidence Medical Education (BEME) review that is relevant to your search:

● The educational effects of portfolios on undergraduate student learning: a Best Evidence Medical Education (BEME) systematic review. *Med Teacher* 2009; **31** :282–98.

You appraise the review so that you can be confident in using its conclusions to inform your practice.

Step 1: Framing the question

Free form question

How does the use of portfolios affect student learning in undergraduate (medical and nursing) education?

Structured question

Population	Undergraduates, defined as students following a course of initial training in a particular profession leading to a degree qualification.
Intervention	A 'portfolio', defined as a collection of evidence of student learning, a learning journal or diary, or a combination of these two elements.
Outcomes	Educational outcomes are classified into levels according to a hierarchy, called the modified Kirkpatrick hierarchy, frequently used in medical education. This attempts to capture the impact of educational interventions using the following levels: participation or completion, modification of attitudes or perceptions, modification of knowledge or skills, change in participants' behaviour and change in delivery of care and health outcomes. This review collected information on any reported outcome demonstrating an effect on student learning as a result of using a portfolio. Changes in delivery of care or improvements in patient outcomes are not normally demonstrable outcomes for undergraduate education as students are not responsible for provision of patient care.
Study designs	Primary research studies of all types that assess the effects on learning of use of a portfolio.

> **Question components**
>
> **The population:** A suitable sample of learners
>
> **The interventions:** An educational intervention
>
> **The outcomes:** Changes in perceptions, attitudes, knowledge, skills, behaviour, etc due to interventions.
>
> **The study design:** Ways of conducting research to assess the effect of intervention on outcomes

The reviewers clearly defined their populations, interventions and outcomes but have not limited the review to studies looking at particular outcomes or study designs. They wish to ensure that no relevant studies are missed by prematurely excluding particular outcomes or study designs. Given the variety of educational research designs and the range of effects of portfolios reported anecdotally, you are satisfied that this approach is appropriate.

While the published review includes studies from professions allied to medicine such as dentistry and physiotherapy, this case study will focus solely on medicine and nursing, which have the largest body of available evidence.

Step 2: Identifying the literature

Searches of the educational literature for medicine and allied professions can be challenging. The relevant educational literature is dispersed across many different databases, subject headings vary considerably and classification of articles against subject headings is not always accurate. The use of only subject headings may not reliably find all relevant articles, and therefore free text words also were used. To ensure comprehensive coverage, reviewers searched 10 different databases from their inception and without language restriction, encompassing the literature from educational (ERIC, British and Australian Education Indices), clinical (MEDLINE, EMBASE, CINAHL, BNI) and social sciences (ASSIA, PsycInfo) (Box C6.1). Search terms and synonyms used reflect closely the population and intervention components of the research question and the reviewers used both subject headings and free text (Box C6.2). The reviewers supplemented the electronic searches with hand searches of the reference lists of selected studies.

The relevance of grey literature to educational systematic reviews depends very much on the topic being examined. For this review, the reviewers judged at an early stage that unpublished sources were unlikely to unearth significant papers not found by other methods and that searching of the grey literature would

---

Box C6.1 Searching for medical education literature

Best Evidence Medical Education (BEME) (www.bemecollaboration.org)

A collaboration committed to the promotion of Best Evidence Medical Education through the dissemination and production of systematic reviews of medical education. An additional objective is the creation of a culture of best evidence medical education amongst teachers, institutions and national bodies.

Some important databases of medical education research

(see also Box 2.2)

BNI The British Nursing Index is a nursing and midwifery database, covering over 200 UK journals and other English language titles.

ASSIA Applied Social Sciences Index and Abstracts is an indexing and abstracting database that covers health, social services, psychology, sociology, economics and politics.

ERIC The Education Resources Information Centre, an extensive database of education journals and grey literature relating to education.

BEI The British Education Index, covering Education Journals, on-line documents and conferences.

AUEI The Australian Education Index, a subscription database consisting of more than 130 000 documents relating to educational research, policy and practice

TIMELIT Topics in Medical Education, a database covering professional education, health education and patient education.

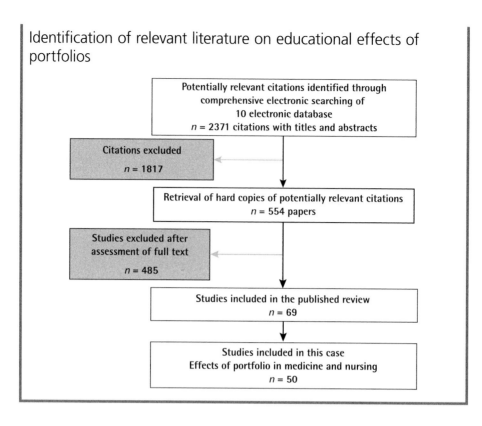

Identification of relevant literature on educational effects of portfolios

Potentially relevant citations identified through comprehensive electronic searching of 10 electronic database
n = 2371 citations with titles and abstracts

Citations excluded
n = 1817

Retrieval of hard copies of potentially relevant citations
n = 554 papers

Studies excluded after assessment of full text
n = 485

Studies included in the published review
n = 69

Studies included in this case
Effects of portfolio in medicine and nursing
n = 50

be a poor use of their valuable time and resources. Whilst this approach may be appropriate in this case, other reviews may require search of the grey literature.

Screening of the 2371 possible citations identified 580 as possibly relevant using predefined selection criteria based on the review question. Of these, full papers of 554 were obtained. Further screening of full manuscripts against selection criteria identified 69 studies for inclusion, 18 from medicine, 32 from nursing and 19 from other professions (Box C6.1). Selection

Box C6.2 How to develop a search term combination for searching electronic bibliographic databases

An example of a search term combination for MEDLINE database

Free form question: How does the use of portfolios affect student learning in undergraduate (medical and nursing) education?

Structured question (not all components may be needed for searching)

- The population   Undergraduate medical and nursing education
- The interventions   Portfolio
- The outcome   Any (not used in search term combination)
- The study design   Any (not used in search term combination)

Question components and relevant search terms	Type of terms		Boolean operator
	MeSH	Free	
The population: Undergraduates			
1 students	x		
2 freshers		x	
3 freshman/men		x	
4 Sophomore		x	OR (captures *population*)
5 Senior		x	
6 additional terms (see in original report of the review)			
7 OR 1-6			
The population: medical education			
8 medical education, undergraduate	x		
9 clinical skills	x		
10 allied health	x		
11 nursing	x		
12 pharmacology	x		OR (captures *population*)
13 medical		x	
14 clinical teaching		x	
15 additional terms (see in original report of the review)			
16 OR 8-15			
The intervention: Portfolio			
17 portfolio		x	
18 learning record		x	
19 case folder		x	
20 case notes		x	
21 learning journal		x	OR (captures *intervention*)
22 log book		x	
23 self reflection		x	
24 additional terms (see in original report of the review)			
25 OR 17-24			
26 **AND /7,16,25**			AND (combines all components)

See related section in Step 2

criteria were established *a priori* and applied by two independent reviewers. Reasons for exclusion were primarily that a particular intervention did not meet the definition of a portfolio or that the study did not contain primary research data.

Aware of the particular factors relating to educational literature, you agree that the reviewers' approach to searching and selection is appropriate and, as far as possible, avoids the risk of missing studies due to publication bias.

Step 3: Assessing study quality

Among the 18 studies in medicine there were two with a comparative design, including one randomized trial, and 16 observational studies without a comparison group. Among the 32 nursing studies there were also two with a comparative design but without randomization, and 29 observational studies without a comparison group. Whilst many studies used a combination of methods, over half of all included studies administered questionnaires to learners; a third used focus group interviews of learners and another third performed direct assessment of portfolios. For educational studies, assessment of study quality is a controversial area, with conflicting views on the appropriateness of particular quality assessment tools. Here, the reviewers assembled a quality checklist and applied this to all studies, regardless of design. In many included studies, it was not possible to make a judgement about study quality due to lack of clarity in reporting. As an example, Box C6.3 illustrates data for four of the 11 quality items used. The reviewers call, as do other commentators on educational research, for authors to report their methods more thoroughly. However, the review also reported an encouraging trend: in each professional group (medicine and nursing) more recent studies had significantly higher quality scores than those

> **Triangulation** is the application and combination of several research methodologies in the study of the same phenomenon.

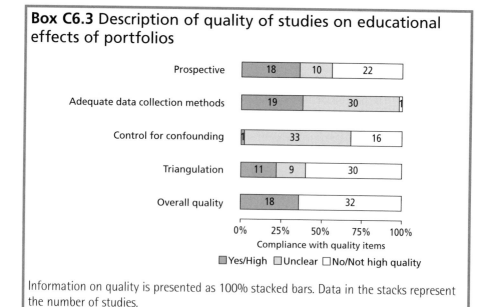

Box C6.3 Description of quality of studies on educational effects of portfolios

Prospective	18 / 10 / 22	
Adequate data collection methods	19 / 30 / 1	
Control for confounding	1 / 33 / 16	
Triangulation	11 / 9 / 30	
Overall quality	18 / 32	

0% 25% 50% 75% 100%
Compliance with quality items
■ Yes/High □ Unclear □ No/Not high quality

Information on quality is presented as 100% stacked bars. Data in the stacks represent the number of studies.

published earlier (data not shown). Overall, 18 of the 50 studies included in the review are classed as higher quality, meeting seven or more of the 11 quality items. The higher quality group included one randomized controlled trial, in which medical students taking a clinical oncology module were randomly allocated to either receive a portfolio or to a control group without a portfolio. The portfolio group recorded patient encounters and received tutorial support in portfolio development.

Step 4: Summarizing the evidence

For this review, as for many other educational systematic reviews, the limitations of the available data meant that meta-analysis of data and statistical investigation of heterogeneity in effects between studies was inappropriate and that a descriptive approach to summarizing the evidence was needed. The reviewers adopted a two-fold approach to this.

First, the reviewers describe how portfolios are generally used in undergraduate education (Box C3.9). Portfolios were mainly used in the clinical setting and their completion was compulsory for students. They required the students to reflect on their learning and share their reflections with other students and staff. In general, students had only limited choice of content and were assessed on their work. Learning journals or diaries were common in nursing, with 'hybrid' portfolios that combined collections of evidence with a learning journal more common in medicine.

Second, the reviewers identify the main messages emerging from the 'higher quality' studies, providing the reader with a rich description of the findings of these studies, grouped according to theme. Higher quality studies reported that using a portfolio can enhance students' knowledge and understanding, particularly their ability to integrate theory with practice, but that these improvements do not always translate into improved assessments. Similarly, portfolios can encourage self-awareness and reflection, but do not guarantee the quality of those reflections. Completing a portfolio can help some students to cope with difficult or uncertain situations, such as a patient death and can prepare them for the rigours of postgraduate training. Engaging with students through a portfolio can help tutors become more aware of students' learning needs, influencing their teaching approaches and allowing them to give more structured feedback. Higher quality studies identified the time required for completion as the main drawback to portfolios. In some cases, where this detracts from other clinical learning, this is not desirable.

The effect of an educational intervention can be assessed using the Kirkpatrick hierarchy as modified for use in educational settings (Box C6.4). The hierarchy classifies the impact studies can have according to the results they demonstrate for various outcomes. Participants'

Box C6.4 Educational outcomes among studies of portfolios

Key themes recorded in higher quality studies. Portfolios may:

- Improve students' knowledge and understanding, especially their ability to integrate theory with practice. However, these effects may not always translate into higher scores in formal assessments
- Encourage students' self-awareness and reflection. However, keeping a portfolio will not, in itself, guarantee the *quality* of those reflections
- Assist tutors in providing structured feedback to their students and increase their awareness of students' needs
- Provide emotional support for students facing difficult situations such as a patient death
- Prepare students for the demands of postgraduate training
- Detract from other clinical learning, if implemented in such a way that the time required for completion is disproportionate.

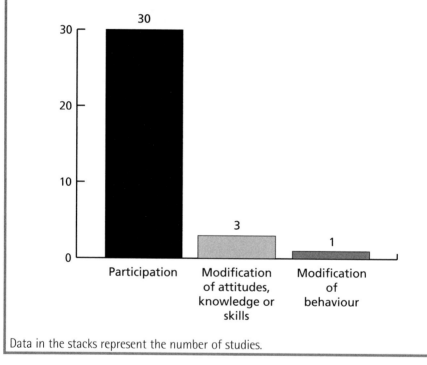

Data in the stacks represent the number of studies.

reactions to an intervention demonstrate impact at a lower level, whilst directly measurable changes in participants' knowledge, skills or behaviours demonstrate impact at a higher level. At the highest level are changes in organizational practice or benefits to patients in terms of improved health outcomes. In this review, most studies demonstrated improvements at lower levels on the Kirkpatrick scale, with only one study (from nursing) reporting a change in participant behaviour.

Step 5: Interpreting the findings

This review showed that the available evidence for the educational effects of portfolios on student learning is limited. Relatively few studies were of higher methodological quality and almost none reported results of outcomes at the higher levels of the modified Kirkpatrick hierarchy. However, limited evidence is not synonymous with lack of effectiveness. The summary of the evidence available does suggest that some important benefits in participants' perceptions, knowledge and skills are possible if portfolios are implemented appropriately. The review makes clear that in order to realize the benefits of portfolios, the time demands on both students and tutors should be kept within reasonable limits. They also caution faculty against assuming that a portfolio will automatically develop students' reflective abilities and suggest that additional guidance on how to reflect should accompany any portfolio intervention that aims to develop these skills. Clearly more research is needed, as is greater clarity and thoroughness of reporting, although the trend towards improvements in quality score in more recent publications is encouraging.

Resolution of scenario

You are disappointed, but not surprised that the evidence base for the effectiveness of portfolios is limited, and are encouraged by the clear directions for implementation offered by the higher quality studies. You share the findings with faculty in your department and develop a proposal for implementation that incorporates the recommendations of the reviewers. You decide to include in your proposal a research study that measures directly the educational effects of portfolios, in order to add to the evidence base on the subject.

Case study 7:
Gauging strength of evidence to guide decision making

Katja Suter

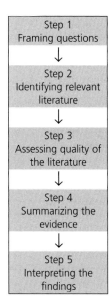

Step 1
Framing questions
↓
Step 2
Identifying relevant literature
↓
Step 3
Assessing quality of the literature
↓
Step 4
Summarizing the evidence
↓
Step 5
Interpreting the findings

Questions arising in patient care can differ from those addressed in research. The quality of studies included in a review can be poor. Their results can be heterogeneous with effects varying from study to study. The effect size summarized in a meta-analysis can be small. Step 5 provided guidance on how to take all this information into account when gauging the strength of the evidence in a systematic review. When does evidence from randomized trials slump to a low strength level? When does evidence from observational studies rise to a moderate or even high strength level? This case study (and Case study 8) illustrates with a worked example how to assess the strength of the evidence collated in a review.

Clinicians often puzzle over the relative benefits and harm of the different classes of drugs for treating the same diagnosis. In hypertension large trials have investigated the effects of angiotensin-receptor blockers (ARBs) *versus* placebo and those of angiotensin-converting-enzyme inhibitors (ACE-Is) *versus* placebo. Based on a published review, this case study explores how to determine the strength of the evidence about the relative benefits of these antihypertensive agents (and Case study 8 explores their adverse effects). It explains how healthcare providers and patients can take this into account when deciding on treatment.

The **quality** of a study depends on the degree to which its design, conduct and analysis minimizes **biases**.

Effect is a measure of association between an *intervention* or *exposure* and an *outcome*.

Heterogeneity is the variation of effects between studies. It may arise because of differences in key characteristics of their *populations*, *interventions* and *outcomes* (clinical heterogeneity), or their study *designs* and quality (methodological heterogeneity).

Scenario: The comparative effectiveness of angiotensin-receptor blockers (ARBs) *versus* angiotensin-converting-enzyme inhibitors (ACE-Is)

You are a general practitioner caring for a 50-year-old overweight patient with recently diagnosed hypertension (150/100 mmHg). His blood pressure did not improve under initial management encouraging him to lose weight. The patient and you decide to start an antihypertensive drug. Among the many drugs recommended as first-line treatment in guidelines, you have a personal preference for renin-system inhibitors. Both drug classes, ARBs and ACE-Is, are effective in lowering blood pressure and preventing major events such as heart attacks and strokes in trials comparing them to placebo. However, you are less certain as to what extent the two drugs differ in their effectiveness when directly compared to each other. This problem has turned up repeatedly in daily practice. Is there a review summarizing the evidence to allow one to establish a preference for one or the other drug?

In a search of MEDLINE using PubMed Clinical Queries at http://www.ncbi.nlm.nih.gov/corehtml/query/static/clinical.shtml (accessed May 2011) you enter "angiotensin-receptor blockers" AND "ACE Inhibitors" AND "Hypertension" in the search box of the Systematic Review feature and click the 'Go' button. The search revealed the following reference:

- Systematic review: comparative effectiveness of angiotensin-converting enzyme inhibitors and angiotensin II receptor blockers for treating essential hypertension. *Ann Intern Med* 2008; **148**: 16-29

A comprehensive report of this review is published by the American Agency for Healthcare Research and Quality (AHRQ) at http://effectivehealthcare.ahrq.gov/repFiles/ACEI_ARBFullReport.pdf (accessed May 2011).

Step 1: Framing the question

Free form question

Which renin-system inhibitor is better in treating hypertension – an ARB or an ACE-inhibitor?

Structured question

The populations	Adult patients with essential hypertension, with or without additional co-morbidities such as diabetes mellitus or established cardiovascular disease.
The interventions	All drugs from the class of ARBs (e.g. losartan, irbesartan, valsartan or telmisartan) compared directly to drugs from the class of ACE inhibitors (e.g. captopril, enalapril, ramipril, or fosinopril) and minimal study duration of 12 weeks.
The outcomes	Mortality, morbidity (stroke, myocardial infarction, heart failure, end-stage renal disease, severe peripheral vascular disease), quality of life and successful monotherapy (Box C7.1).
The study designs	All randomized controlled trials.

Guidelines are systematically developed statements to assist practitioners and patients in making decisions about specific clinical situations. Their recommendations should reflect the strength of the underpinning evidence.

Question components

The population: A clinically suitable sample of patients

The interventions: Comparison of groups with different interventions

The outcomes: Changes in health state due to interventions

The study design: Ways of conducting research to assess the effect of interventions (Box 1.4)

Surrogate outcome measurements substitute for direct measures of how patients feel, what their function is, or if they survive. They include physiological variables or measures of subclinical disease. To be valid, the surrogate must be statistically correlated with the clinically relevant outcome.

Box C7.1 Hierarchy of outcomes in antihypertensive therapy ranked by importance and directness of measurement

Importance*	Direct measurement (descending order of importance)	Surrogate measurement
Critical	**Reduce mortality** • All-cause mortality • Cardiovascular mortality • Cerebrovascular mortality **Reduce major morbidity** • Disabling stroke • Myocardial infarction • Moderate to severe heart failure • Advanced or end-stage renal disease • Leg ulceration and amputation due to peripheral vascular disease	Physiological variables or disease markers which only indirectly capture the outcome • Lipid levels • Function of glucose metabolism as markers of diabetes and diabetes control: blood glucose, glycosylated haemoglobin HbA1c
Important	**Reduce mild morbidity** • Mild angina pectoris • Mild intermittent claudication • Mild renal impairment • Transient ischaemic attack **Improve quality of life** (QoL) • General QoL • Specific dimensions of health-related QoL (e.g. cognitive function, symptomatic well-being) • Disease-specific QoL **Successful monotherapy**	• Left ventricular function • Renal function as marker of renal disease: serum creatinine, glomerular filtration rate
Less important	**Reduce cost** • Reduction in drug cost to the healthcare system (policy makers might call this an important or critical outcome)	

This expands on the question posed in Boxes 1.2 and 1.3
Also see Box C8.1

* Importance of outcome coded in different shades of grey for ease of display. Ranking of importance outcomes can be undertaken through formal survey of patients or practitioners asking them to provide responses on a scale anchored between critical at one extreme and not at all important at the other. An explicit approach enables users of a review to compare published judgements with the judgements relevant for their own environment.

When thinking about outcomes, one needs to consider all outcomes that are important to patients. Most outcomes belong to one of three broad categories: mortality, morbidity and quality of life. Mortality can be separated into all-cause mortality or disease-specific (e.g. cardio- or cerebro-vascular) mortality. Morbidity addresses, for example, stroke, myocardial infarction, heart failure, end-stage renal disease or severe peripheral vascular disease. Quality of life can refer to general quality of life assessed with generic instruments or specific dimensions, like physical function, pain or sleep. Patients consider successful monotherapy as an important outcome as it prevents them being exposed to an additional drug, avoiding potential adverse effects.

Some outcomes are more important to patients than others. Whether an outcome is critical, important or less important also depends on the perspective. Cost might be of little importance to patients when their drugs are fully covered by their health insurance. It might be important or even critical from the perspective of a policy maker. Reviewers should therefore indicate whose perspective they take. Often research focuses on intermediate or surrogate measures of outcomes such as control of blood pressure, lipids, glomerular filtration rate or blood glucose. Surrogate measurements do not capture outcomes directly. This indirectness should be taken into account when assigning a level of strength to the evidence.

The reviewers had a well-founded concern that no studies might exist for some of the clinically relevant outcomes. They therefore included surrogate outcome measurements such as impaired glomerular filtration rate for end-stage renal disease. Clinicians and decision makers would need to extrapolate from such a surrogate marker. Uncertainty through indirectness lowers the strength of the evidence. The large licensing studies comparing ARBs and ACE-Is against placebo or other antihypertensive agents evaluated only surrogate outcomes. The review on which this case study is based deals with the issue of indirectness head on. For illustrative purposes, this chapter confines itself to assessing three outcomes: mortality and major cardiovascular morbidity, end-stage renal disease and successful monotherapy for blood pressure control.

Step 2: Identifying the relevant literature

An electronic search was undertaken in two databases, in PubMed/ MEDLINE and in CENTRAL, the Cochrane Central Register of Controlled Trials (Box 2.2). Furthermore, the reviewers had access to the register of the Cochrane Hypertension Review Group. Their search terms included hypertension (*population*), drug *interventions* and *study designs*, but did not specify *outcomes*. The results were limited to studies published in the English language

Clinically relevant outcome measurements directly measure how patients feel, what their function is, or if they survive.

Strength of evidence describes the extent to which we can be confident that the estimate of an observed effect is correct for important questions. It takes into account directness of outcome measure, study design, study quality, heterogeneity, imprecision and publication bias (this is not an exhaustive list).

Identifying relevant literature
- Develop search term combinations
- Search relevant electronic databases
- Search other relevant resources
- Obtain full papers of potentially relevant citations
- Include/exclude studies using pre-set selection criteria
- Assess for risk of missing studies

after the year 1988. The researchers used additional material that five pharmaceutical companies submitted to the AHRQ. They reviewed reference lists of relevant review articles, and citations identified by a peer reviewer of their protocol. Box C7.2 documents the selection process: The review finally included 45 randomized trials. A funnel plot explored the risk of missing studies (see Box C7.5).

Box C7.2 Identification of relevant literature on the comparative effectiveness of angiotensin-receptor blockers (ARBs) *versus* angiotensin-converting-enzyme inhibitors (ACE-Is)

Electronic databases searched

1. MEDLINE
2. Cochrane Central Register of Controlled Trials
3. Register of the Cochrane Hypertension Review Group

Study identification flow chart

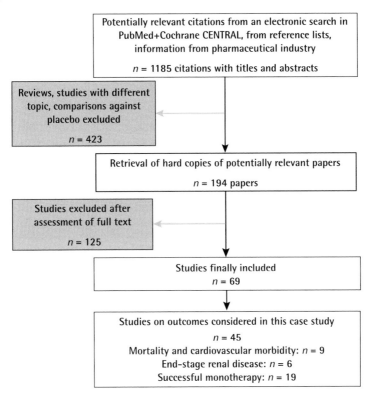

This case study only describes the evidence for three outcomes.

Step 3: Assessing study quality

Study design threshold for study selection

The reviewers, concerned that they might not find enough randomized trials, accepted a low threshold for study design by including observational studies with a comparison group. They considered randomized and non-randomized controlled trials, prospective and retrospective cohort and case-control studies. The decision ensured that they could fall back on observational data in case of insufficient data from randomized studies. This case study will only consider the results from the randomized trials included.

Description of study quality assessment for the selected trials

The checklist for methodological quality of the studies addresses generic and specific quality items (Box C7.3). For key generic biases, it explored whether randomization (including allocation concealment) was appropriate, whether the studies blinded patients, healthcare providers and outcome assessors, and whether

The **quality** of a study depends on the degree to which its design, conduct and analysis minimizes **biases**.

Bias either exaggerates or underestimates the 'true' effect of an *intervention*.

The **direction of effect** indicates a beneficial or a harmful effect. The point estimate of effect tells us about direction and magnitude of effect.

Box C7.3 Description of study quality on the comparative effectiveness of angiotensin-receptor blockers (ARBs) *versus* angiotensin-converting-enzyme inhibitors (ACE-Is) in essential hypertension.

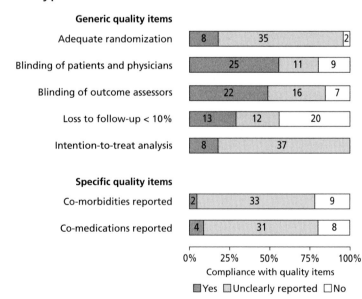

Information on quality is presented as 100% stacked bars. Data in the stacks represent the numbers of the studies.

the groups remained comparable throughout the observation period by assessing cross-over, losses to follow-up and potential differentials between the groups. It checked whether the analysis included all patients as randomized (intention-to-treat analysis). Specific quality items comprise equal distribution of co-morbidities such as diabetes or renal disease and co-interventions such as concomitant treatment with additional antihypertensive drugs or dose-escalating protocols among both treatment arms.

As shown in Box C7.3 most studies had at least some methodological weaknesses or lacked unambiguous reporting. This applied in particular to adequacy of randomization, completeness of follow-up and execution of an intention-to-treat analysis. Half the studies blinded patients, physicians and outcome assessors. The assessment of the specific quality items found insufficient reporting about co-morbid conditions of the patients and about concurrent medication. These limitations lower the methodological quality of the individual studies, introducing a risk of bias.

Step 4: Summarizing the evidence

Heterogeneity of the results across studies, precision of the observed effects and the likelihood of publication bias play a role in gauging the strength of the evidence.

Mortality and major cardiovascular morbidity

Only nine of the 45 included randomized studies reported at least one of the outcomes (mortality, stroke, myocardial infarction or heart failure), and only five of those nine studies observed at least one event (Box C7.4). Most studies followed the patients up only short term (median 6 months; range 3.5–60 months). One study with the longest follow-up contributed 55 of the 61 events (90%) across all studies and all interventions. Despite the inclusion of more than 3000 patients there was imprecision because only very few events were captured. As an example, the four studies with 1628 patients detected only 17 events of a myocardial infarction. The scarcity of events in outcomes led to wide confidence intervals. There was no particular heterogeneity of results. Overall, the findings were compatible with superiority or inferiority of either drug.

End-stage renal disease

Six studies assessed renal function (i.e. the capacity of the kidney to remove metabolites from the body) using different measures such as serum creatinine, glomerular filtration rate or creatinine clearance (Box C7.4). To collate different measures into a single summary estimate of renal function requires conversion to standardized difference in means or SMD. On this measure, a minus value indicates that the ACE-Is were superior and a plus

The **precision of effect** relates to the degree of uncertainty in the estimation of effect that is due to the play of chance. The confidence interval tells us about precision.

Point estimate of effect is its observed value in a study.

Confidence interval is the imprecision in the point estimate, i.e. the range around it within which the 'true' value of the effect can be expected to lie with a given degree of certainty (e.g. 95%).

Point estimate

Confidence interval

Standardized difference in means or SMD is an effect measure for continuous data where studies have measured an outcome using different scales (e.g. pain may be measured in a variety of ways or depression assessed on a variety of scales). In order to summarize such studies, it is necessary to standardize the results into a uniform scale.

Box C7.4 Results for death, major cardiovascular and renal outcomes among randomized trials comparing angiotensin-receptor blockers (ARBs) *versus* angiotensin-converting-enzyme inhibitors (ACE-Is)

Outcome: Mortality and major cardiovascular morbidity

Outcome	Number of studies, patients, events	Relative risk[+] (ACE/ACE-I)	95% CI	Heterogeneity Chi^2/I^2-test
Mortality	8 studies, 4264 patients, 15 events	1.05	0.40 to 2.75	$p = 0.79$/0%
Stroke	3 studies, 1779 patients, 13 events	0.84	0.30 to 2.35	$p = 0.56$/0%
Myocardial infarction	4 studies, 1628 patients, 17 events	1.32	0.54 to 3.57	$p = 0.61$/0%
Heart failure	1 study, 168 patients, 16 events	1.20	0.68 to 1.78	Not relevant

Outcome: End-stage renal disease

Study	Surrogate measurement of renal function*	Patients (total)	Follow–up (months)	SMD[$]	95% CI
1	GFR (ml/min)	96	36	0.27	−0.29 to 0.83
2	CCl (ml/min)	29	4.25	0.55	−0.19 to 1.29
3	CCl (ml/min)	33	6	−0.57	−1.34 to 0.21
4	S-creatinine (mg/dl)	57	12	0.38	−0.23 to 0.99
5	S-creatinine (mg/dl)	89	3	0.00	−0.43 to 0.43
6	GFR (ml/min)	250	60	−0.12	−0.38 to 0.15
	Pooled estimate		*Random effects model*	*0.05*	*−0.20 to 0.30*

[+] *A relative risk > 1 indicated that the ACE-Is were superior, a relative risk < 1 indicated that the ARBs were superior.*

[$] *SMD = Standardized difference in means*

* *Surrogate measurements: CCl = creatinine clearance; GFR = glomerular filtration rate; S-creatinine = serum creatinine*

Also see Box C7.1 for importance of outcomes.

value indicates that the ARBs were superior; zero indicated the line of no effect. There was no particular heterogeneity of results from study to study. Pooling the results of the individual studies using a random effects model shows a negligible effect, the SMD of 0.05 favouring ARBs. The 95% confidence interval of −0.20–0.30 confirmed that there was no difference in effect between the two drugs, and that the data would be compatible with both superiority and inferiority of either drug.

Relative risk (RR) is an effect measure for binary data. It is the ratio of risk in the experimental group to the risk in the control group.

Successful monotherapy

Nineteen trials evaluated the potency of either drug in controlling blood pressure to allow monotherapy for treating hypertension, and potentially improving compliance. The forest plot in Box C7.5 displays the results of the individual studies. There was no particular heterogeneity of results from study to study. The summary estimate expressed as risk difference did not detect any difference between ARBs and ACE-Is, and the narrow 95% confidence interval of −0.02–0.02 confirmed that a difference did not exist.

Publication bias could only be reliably assessed for this outcome. A funnel plot explored the risk for missing studies. The search for primary studies had only covered two electronic databases. One of these, CENTRAL, contained citations of trials from a range of bibliographic databases, notably MEDLINE (around 60% of the records) and EMBASE, from other published and unpublished sources, as well as from hand-searching journals in non-English languages. Screening the reference lists of existing reviews contributed additional references, as did the public reviewing the draft review protocol and materials from pharmaceutical companies. Visual inspection of the large number of studies for the outcome successful monotherapy in a funnel plot did not raise suspicion about truncation, reducing concern about the risk of publication bias (Box C7.5).

> **Risk difference (RD)** is an effect measure for binary data. In a comparative study, it is the difference in event rates between two groups.

Box C7.5 Forest and funnel plots for successful monotherapy among trials comparing angiotensin-receptor blockers (ARBs) *versus* angiotensin-converting-enzyme inhibitors (ACE-Is) in essential hypertension

Forest plot

Study or Subgroup	ARB Events	ARB Total	ACE-I Events	ACE-I Total	Weight	Risk Difference Random, 95%CI	Risk Difference Random, 95%CI
Argenziano 1999	182	264	182	264	8.7%	0.00 [−0.08, 0.08]	
Cuspidi 2002	53	115	57	124	3.4%	0.00 [−0.13, 0.13]	
Eguchi 2003	29	37	29	36	1.6%	−0.02 [−0.21, 0.16]	
Forgari 2004	45	75	39	75	2.2%	0.08 [−0.08, 0.24]	
Ghiadoni 2003	23	29	21	28	1.1%	0.04 [−0.17, 0.26]	
Karlberg 1999	89	139	88	139	4.2%	0.01 [−0.11, 0.12]	
Kavgaci 2002	13	20	7	10	0.4%	−0.05 [−0.40, 0.30]	
Lacourciere 2000	20	52	30	51	1.5%	−0.20 [−0.39, −0.01]	
LaRochelle 1997	11	121	4	61	8.4%	0.03 [−0.06, 0.11]	
Malacco 2004	479	604	479	609	25.8%	0.01 [−0.04, 0.05]	
Mogensen 2000	54	66	46	64	2.6%	0.10 [−0.04, 0.24]	
Neutel 1999	169	385	93	193	7.3%	−0.04 [−0.13, 0.04]	
Robles 2004	10	15	11	15	0.5%	−0.07 [−0.39, 0.26]	
Rosei 2005	39	66	40	63	1.9%	−0.04 [−0.21, 0.12]	
Ruff 1996	3	50	4	25	2.2%	−0.10 [−0.26, 0.06]	
Ruilope 2001	153	168	152	163	16.2%	−0.02 [−0.08, 0.04]	
Saito 2004	66	200	51	214	7.2%	0.09 [0.01, 0.10]	
Townsend 1995	62	132	72	136	3.8%	−0.06 [−0.18, 0.06]	
Uchiyama–Tanaka 2005	14	18	19	25	0.8%	−0.02 [−0.24, 0.27]	
Total (95% CI)		**2556**		**2295**	**100%**	**−0.00 [−0.02, 0.02]**	

Heterogeneity: Tau² = 0.00; Chi² = 16.76, df= 18 (P = 0.54); I² = 0%
Test for overall effect: Z = 0.02 (P = 0.99)

−0.5

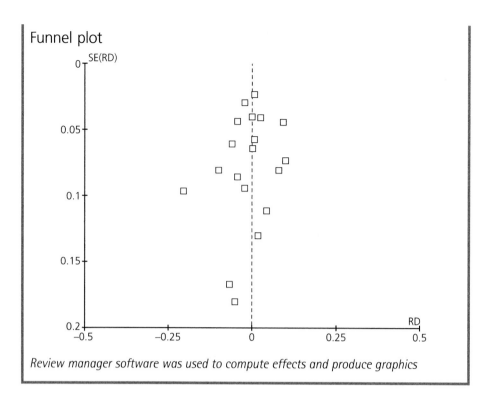

Funnel plot

Review manager software was used to compute effects and produce graphics

Step 5: Interpreting the findings

Before moving on to gauging the strength of the evidence, the key findings concerning importance of outcomes and precision of results are tabulated (Box C7.6). These are put together with study design, methodological limitations in study quality, inconsistency of results and risk of publication bias to assign a level of strength to the evidence (Box C7.7).

The strength level first assigned to the evidence on the outcome mortality and major cardiovascular morbidity is high as it emanates from randomized design. This initial assignment is re-adjusted as the strength is limited by the risk of bias due to methodological limitations and imprecision related to the scarcity of events. Each shortcoming justifies reduction in the strength level initially assigned. Consistency in results reassures that effects do not vary between high and lower quality studies. This indicates that methodological limitations did not exert an impact on the effect sizes. It may be judged that the overall strength of the evidence is relegated finally to a low level, which means that our confidence in the observed effect of the two drugs on mortality and cardiovascular morbidity is limited and the 'true' effect may be substantially different.

The second critical outcome, end-stage renal disease due to hypertension, is measured using surrogates. Limitations through indirectness, risk of bias and imprecision of the effect are serious. Thus the initially assigned high level, due to randomized dosing,

The Grading of Recommendations Assessment, Development and Evaluation (**GRADE**) working group is an informal collaboration that aims to develop a comprehensive methodology for assessing the strength of the evidence collated in systematic reviews and for generating recommendations from evidence in guidelines. See www. gradeworkinggroup. org. Interpretation of findings in this case study draws on this methodology.

may be relegated to very low strength of evidence. This indicates that the 'true' effect on end-stage renal disease is likely to be substantially different from the observed effect renal function.

The third outcome, successful monotherapy, is important to patients. These studies also have methodological limitations. The large numbers of events produce a narrow confidence interval around the point estimate of effect. There is no evidence of risk of publication bias. Thus, on balance, the high level of the strength initially assigned on account of randomized design is lowered to moderate strength of evidence. Hence, this evidence is likely to represent the 'true' effect.

Resolution of the scenario

The verdict, taking into account the overall strength of the evidence is transparent: Head-to-head comparison of the two drugs did not show a convincing difference in effect across a range of critical and important outcomes. While one cannot be absolutely certain that differences in effect do not exist for some outcome measures, the appraised evidence does not provide strong clues for the existence of a difference. Stronger evidence on critical and important outcomes would be desirable, though in practice the appraised evidence is reassuring. One could consider prescribing one or another agent on account of benefits being similar. A key element impinging on this decision is consideration of the risk of potential adverse effects. Case study 8 will explore this issue.

Box C7.6 Summary of findings of a review comparing angiotensin-receptor blockers (ARBs) *versus* angiotensin-converting-enzyme inhibitors (ACE-Is) in essential hypertension

Importance	Outcome	Measurement	Number of patients		Summary effect Effect [95% CI]
			ARB	ACE-I	Relative risk (ARB/ACE-I)
Critical	Mortality and major cardiovascular morbidity 9 trials Total events: 61	Mortality	1659	1663	1.05 [0.40 to 2.75]
		Stroke			0.84 [0.30 to 2.35]
		Myocardial infarction			1.32 [0.54 to 3.57]
		Heart failure			1.20 [0.68 to 1.78]
	End stage renal disease 6 trials	Renal function (surrogate)	253	246	Effect size (SMD*) 0.051 [−0.19 to 0.29]
Important	Successful monotherapy 19 trials Total events: 2938	Successful monotherapy	2556	2295	Risk difference (ARB − ACE-I) −0.00 [−0.03 to 0.02]

* SMD = standardized mean difference

Box C7.7 Assessing strength of the evidence collated in a review comparing angiotensin-receptor blockers (ARBs) *versus* angiotensin-converting-enzyme inhibitors (ACE-Is) in essential hypertension

Outcome and its Importance	Study design	Directness of outcome measure	Study quality (risk of bias)	Inconsistency of results (heterogeneity)	Imprecision of effects	Publication bias	Strength of evidence
Mortality and major cardiovascular morbidity	Randomized trial	Direct	Some limitations	Consistent	Imprecise	Not assessed	*Low*
(Critical)	*Initially assigned a high strength level*	→ *No change*	→ *Relegation*	→ *No change*	→ *Relegation*	→ *No change*	⌐
End-stage renal disease	Randomized trial	Indirect	Some limitations	Consistent	Imprecise	Not assessed	*Very low*
(Critical)	*Initially assigned a high strength level*	→ *Relegation*	→ *Relegation*	→ *No change*	→ *Relegation*	→ *No change*	⌐
Successful monotherapy	Randomized trial	Direct	Some limitations	Consistent	Precise	Not detected	*Moderate*
(Important)	*Initially assigned a high strength level*	→ *No change*	→ *Relegation*	→*No change*	→ *No change*	→ *No change*	⌐

● Case study 8: *To use or not to use a therapy? Incorporating evidence on adverse effects*

Katja Suter

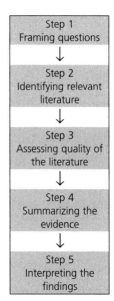

Step 1
Framing questions
↓
Step 2
Identifying relevant literature
↓
Step 3
Assessing quality of the literature
↓
Step 4
Summarizing the evidence
↓
Step 5
Interpreting the findings

For making informed decisions, healthcare professionals and patients need to balance the benefits against the adverse effects of interventions. Systematic reviews of effectiveness should include information on adverse effects and other harms, but the primary studies they include often do not capture data on these outcomes, or only do this secondarily. To allow collation of information on rare harmful outcomes, particularly those that develop over a long time period, systematic reviews need to include a range of study *designs* (see Case study 2). Another issue reviews need to consider is how comprehensive they need to be in the coverage of the potential adverse effects. Package leaflets of drugs or information for the user that accompanies medicinal products often report 50 or more adverse effects of varying frequency and severity. Reviews covering evidence on *all* possible adverse effects are not always necessary or feasible. To narrow the focus on a *few* severe adverse effects that particularly impact on the clinical decision would be reasonable. This will allow weighing up of benefits against potential harms.

Adverse effect is an undesirable and unintended harmful or unpleasant reaction resulting from an *intervention*.

This case study demonstrates how to seek and assess evidence on adverse effects of a drug. It will evaluate potential harms associated with a drug assessed for its effectiveness in Case study 7. Based on a published review, it will apply the review theory related to framing questions, identifying literature, assessing study quality, summarizing the results on adverse effects, and gauging the strength of the evidence on two treatment options, showing how to come up with a decision.

Scenario: Considering adverse effects when choosing an antihypertensive treatment

You are a general practitioner who currently has an overweight 50-year-old patient with recently diagnosed hypertension (150/100 mmHg). The blood pressure did not improve under the initial management strategy of encouraging him to lose weight. Both the patient and you decide to start an antihypertensive medication. Among the many drugs recommended as first-line treatment in guidelines, you favour a renin-system blocking drug, either angiotensin-converting-enzyme inhibitors (ACE-Is) or angiotensin-receptor blockers (ARBs). Which one to choose?

Recently, you critically appraised a systematic review (Case study 7) comparing ARBs with ACE-Is head-to-head, which showed similar effects for ARBs and ACE-Is in reducing blood pressure. The review did not show differences between the ARBs and ACE-Is for outcomes such as death, major cardiovascular morbidity and end-stage renal disease. You want to explore adverse effects, and you consult the following review:

- Systematic review: comparative effectiveness of angiotensin-converting-enzyme inhibitors and angiotensin-II-receptor blockers for treating essential hypertension. *Ann Intern Med* 2008; **148**: 16–29.

A comprehensive report of this review is published by the American Agency for Healthcare Research and Quality (AHRQ) at http://effectivehealthcare.ahrq.gov/repFiles/ACEI_ARBFullReport. pdf (accessed July 2009). The review of adverse effects in this report collates results from randomized trials and observational studies. The assessment of adverse effects captured in randomized trials follows the same principles demonstrated in Case study 7. Frequently, however, observational studies are the only source of information for adverse effects, and this case study demonstrates how to appraise this information. Mind you, if available, one would always consider the evidence on common side-effects from experimental studies, because of the lower risk of bias associated with this design (Box 1.4).

Step 1: Framing the question

Free form question

Is there a difference in adverse effects between ARBs and ACE-Is?

Structured question

The populations   Adults with essential hypertension.

The interventions   All drugs from the class of ARBs (e.g. losartan, irbesartan, valsartan or telmisartan) compared to drugs from the class of ACE-Is (e.g. captopril, enalapril, ramipril or fosinopril) and minimal study duration of 12 weeks.

The outcomes   Key adverse effects including cough, headache, dizziness and 'withdrawal due to adverse events' (this case study focuses on cough and withdrawals only).

The study designs   Experimental and observational studies with a control group (this case study focuses on evidence collated from cohort and case-control studies).

Not all adverse effects have the same impact on decision making. More common and more serious ones that affect the patient's wellbeing weigh heavier than physiological changes without particular consequences or rare adverse effects. Box C8.1 ranks harmful outcomes from ARBs and ACE-Is according to their importance, alongside the beneficial outcomes from Case study 7. One might notice that in Box C8.1 common adverse effects such as increase in serum creatinine, increase in liver enzymes or reduction in haemoglobin are missing. Such changes in physiological variables are surrogate measurements and supply only indirect evidence for drug-related renal failure, hepatitis or symptomatic anaemia respectively. Surrogates lower the strength of the evidence.

How should one select a few key adverse effects from the many potential harms? More common ones tend to play a more significant role in patient care than rare or very rare ones, even if the latter are more serious. (Very) rare effects are less likely to prevent us from recommending a drug. For example, Stevens–Johnson syndrome, a potentially life-threatening drug reaction, occurs in less than 1 in 10000 cases. Considering patient preferences, clinicians would usually not take this low level of risk into account when deciding to prescribe or not to prescribe a drug. For illustrative purposes, this case study is restricted to two adverse outcomes: cough and 'withdrawals due to adverse effects'.

Step 2: Identifying relevant literature

Capturing studies on adverse effects is a challenge. This is because the terminology for adverse effect lacks standardization and adverse effects are usually not listed in the title or abstract. Furthermore, databases like MEDLINE (PubMed) do not have a separate MeSH term for adverse effects, which may exist as a subheading to certain MeSH terms. This improves precision but lowers the sensitivity of a search (Step 2, Sections 2.1.2 and 2.1.3).

The reviewers searched MEDLINE and CENTRAL (Cochrane Central Register of Controlled Trials) for randomized trials and observational studies in the English language and accessed a register of the Cochrane Hypertension Review Group. Box C8.2 shows the search term combinations used for the MEDLINE database. The researchers refrained from defining adverse effects as outcomes in their search strategy, acknowledging their poor coding in electronic databases. The assessment for adverse effects took place during full-text screening.

The search provided 1185 citations, the screening of titles/abstracts narrowed the results down to 194 citations for full-text assessments, the final study pool for the systematic review included 69 reports. Of those, 26 RCTs and three observational studies reported on cough, and 22 RTCs and two observational studies on 'withdrawals due to adverse effects' (Box C8.3).

Withdrawal of participants or patients can be for many reasons, e.g. non-compliance with the intervention, cross-over to an alternative intervention, drop out of the study and loss to follow-up. When the reason for withdrawal is the appearance of an adverse effect, this information can be used as an outcome measure for drug safety.

Sensitivity of a search is the proportion of relevant studies identified by a search strategy expressed as a percentage of all relevant studies on a given topic. It is a measure of the comprehensiveness of a search method. *Do not confuse with sensitivity of a test.*

Precision of a search is the proportion of relevant studies identified by a search strategy. This is expressed as a percentage of all studies (relevant and irrelevant) identified by that strategy. It is a measure of the ability of a search to exclude irrelevant studies. Do not confuse with precision of effect.

Study design filter employs a search term combination to capture citations of studies of a particular design.

Box C8.1 Comparison of beneficial outcomes and adverse effects of antihypertensive treatment with angiotensin-receptor blockers (ARBs) *versus* angiotensin-converting-enzyme inhibitors (ACE-Is)

Importance*	Beneficial outcomes (descending order of importance)	Adverse effects
Critical	**Reduce mortality** • All-cause mortality • Cardiovascular mortality • Cerebrovascular mortality **Reduce major morbidity** • Disabling stroke • Myocardial infarction • Moderate to severe heart failure • Advanced or end-stage renal disease • Leg ulceration and amputation due to peripheral vascular disease	Frequent and non-reversible effects
Important	**Reduce mild morbidity** • Mild angina pectoris • Mild intermittent claudication • Mild renal impairment • Transient ischaemic attack **Improve quality of life** (QoL) • General QoL • Specific dimensions of health related QoL (e.g. cognitive function, symptomatic well-being) • Disease-specific QoL **Successful monotherapy**	Low incidence and fully reversible effects Morbidity • Cough (frequent) • Headache (frequent) • Dizziness (frequent) • Angio-oedema (rare) • Acute renal failure (rare)
Less important	**Reduce cost** • Reduction in drug cost to the healthcare system (policy makers might call this an important or critical outcome)	Very low incidence and fully reversible effects • Dose-dependent change in taste (occasional) • Mild moods swings (occasional) • Hepatitis (very rare) • Symptomatic anaemia (very rare) • Steven-Johnson syndrome (very rare)

* The beneficial outcomes are taken from Case study 7; also see Box C7.1

Adverse effects can occur very frequently (> 1 in 10); frequently (between 1 in 10 and 1 in 100); occasionally (between 1 in 100 and in /1000); rarely (between 1 in 1000 and 1 in 10000); very rarely (<1 in 10000, including singular reports). This scale is only a suggestion.

Box C8.2 Search term combination for Ovid MEDLINE to identify citations of literature on the adverse effects of angiotensin-receptor blockers (ARBs) *versus* angiotensin-converting-enzyme inhibitors (ACE-Is)

The original search term combination consisted of 56 sets of terms, where of the following table shows a selection to give an example how to combine search terms.

Question components and a selection of relevant terms	Type of terms Free	Type of terms MeSH	Boolean operator (*see glossary*)
The population: Patients with hypertension			
1. exp hypertension/		x	
2. *additional terms (see in original report of the review)*			OR (captures *population*)
3. or/1–2			
The interventions: ARBs and ACE-Is			
4. (losartan OR valsartan).tw	x		
5. angiotensin II type 1 receptor blockers/		x	
6. (quinapril OR captopril OR enalapril).tw	x		
7. angiotensin-converting-enzyme inhibitors/		x	OR (captures *intervention*)
8. *additional terms (see in original report of the review)*			
9. or/4–8			
The Outcomes			
No search is performed to capture *outcomes*			
10. and/3,9			AND (combines *population* and *intervention*)
The study designs: Observational studies			
11. Comparative Study/		x	
12. exp Evaluation Studies/		x	
13. Follow-up Studies/		x	
14. (control$ OR prospective$ OR volunteers$).tw.	x		OR (captures *study designs*)
15. *additional terms (see in original report of the review)*			
16. or/11–15			
17. and/10, 16			AND (combines *population* and *intervention* and *study designs*)
18. limit 16 to human			

Box C8.3 Identification of relevant literature on adverse effects of angiotensin-receptor blockers (ARBs) *versus* angiotensin-converting-enzyme inhibitors (ACE-Is)

Electronic databases searched

1. MEDLINE
2. Cochrane Central Register of Controlled Trials
3. Register of the Cochrane Hypertension Review Group

Study identification flow chart

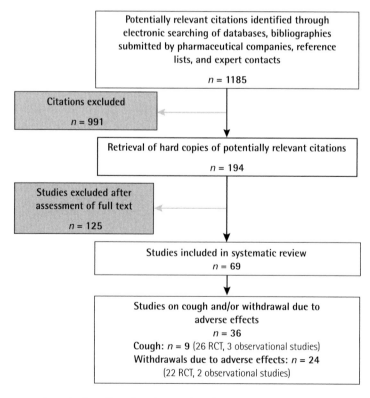

Potentially relevant citations identified through electronic searching of databases, bibliographies submitted by pharmaceutical companies, reference lists, and expert contacts
n = 1185

Citations excluded
n = 991

Retrieval of hard copies of potentially relevant citations
n = 194

Studies excluded after assessment of full text
n = 125

Studies included in systematic review
n = 69

Studies on cough and/or withdrawal due to adverse effects
n = 36
Cough: *n* = 9 (26 RCT, 3 observational studies)
Withdrawals due to adverse effects: *n* = 24
(22 RCT, 2 observational studies)

* This case study only describes the observational studies in detail.

Step 3: Assessing study quality

Study design threshold for study selection

Different study *designs* need to be considered for information about adverse effects. Randomized trials are well suited for common, anticipated adverse effects, whereas observational studies may be more useful for delayed or rare adverse effects. In the latter situation, it will be reasonable to consider more than one observational design, taking into account the strengths and weaknesses of each (Box 1.4). The review underlying this case study included randomized trials and observational (cohort and case-control) studies. This case study demonstrates how to appraise observational evidence.

Quality assessment of observational studies on safety

Quality assessment of observational studies is concerned with methodological issues similar to those relevant for randomized studies (Step 3, Box 3.2). Establishing comparable groups to prevent selection bias, ensuring appropriate use of the *interventions*, minimizing bias in the measurement of *outcomes*, and an appropriate statistical analysis are key to study quality. The key quality items used in this case study are described below:

Prospective design: A prospective design with forward planning, comprehensive assessment of the patients and collection of all relevant data may facilitate efforts outlined above to minimize bias (Box C2.2). One might have access to a database which has already meticulously documented the enrolment of patients, carefully measured a wide variety of prognostic factors, follow-up all patients and rigorously recorded their outcomes. In this situation a retrospective design will not be a particular disadvantage. A prospective study, badly done, may fail to document how patients were selected, measure prognostic factors in an incomplete and sloppy way, and lose a large proportion of their patients to follow-up. Therefore, prospective or retrospective should not be treated as quality criteria in themselves. In addition, one should look to see whether studies adhered to the criteria listed above.

Assembling comparable groups at the outset: Groups that are unequal in important prognostic factors pose a major threat to the validity of observational studies. This is because those differences – rather than the differences in the interventions – may be linked to the outcomes. (Large) experimental studies balance out potential confounding factors by randomly allocating patients with varying risks factors equally between groups. Assembling groups that are similar at baseline is more challenging in observational studies, and most of the time they rely on the analysis to perform statistical adjustment for group differences.

The **quality** of a study depends on the degree to which its design, conduct and analysis minimizes **biases**.

Bias either exaggerates or underestimates the 'true' effect of an *intervention*.

Confounding is a situation in comparative studies where the effect of an *exposure* or *intervention* on an *outcome* is distorted due to the association of the *outcome* with another factor, which can prevent or cause the *outcome* independent of the *exposure* or *intervention*. Data analysis may be adjusted for confounding in observational studies.

To do so, the researchers have to identify at baseline all relevant prognostic factors and co-morbidities that can bring about 'adverse effects' regardless of the *exposure*; avoiding ACE-Is in patients with chronic bronchitis as cough may be an adverse effect of ACE-I. This selective prescribing behaviour could bias the assessment of frequency of cough.

Ascertaining exposure: In observational studies it is essential to correctly identify those exposed and those not exposed to an intervention. Consider a study that included new and current users of antihypertensive drugs. More 'new users' of antihypertensive drugs were in the ACE-I group, while more 'previous users' of antihypertensive drugs entered the ARB group. A considerable proportion of those 'previous users' had experienced cough using ACE-Is and had switched to ARBs before entering the study. This could reduce the frequency of cough associated with ACE-Is. Thus it is important to minimize misclassification in exposure, by collecting information on all co-medications and any cross-over of medications.

Outcome ascertainment: Outcome assessment in observational studies is vulnerable to the same biases as in experimental studies. Measurement bias has to be dealt with using similar precautions. Subjective outcomes such as a bothersome cough or the experience of adverse effects that warranted withdrawal demand the person ascertaining the outcome be kept blind to the *exposure* status. Only few observational studies manage to implement appropriate measures to achieve blinding. Adverse effects with less frequent or delayed occurrence need a (sufficiently) long follow-up for detection.

Appropriate analysis: Once key relevant prognostic factors have been identified, appropriate adjustment in the analysis for differences of those factors between the groups increases the chance that any observed association between *exposure* and *outcome* reflects the 'truth'. It is often difficult to identify and adjust for *all* confounding factors. Loss to follow-up and missing values interfere with performing an appropriate analysis.

> **Prognosis** is a probable course or outcome of a disease. **Prognostic factors** are patient or disease characteristics that influence the course. Good prognosis is associated with a low rate of undesirable outcomes. Poor prognosis is associated with a high rate of undesirable outcomes.

Description of quality of the selected observational studies

A separate description of quality assessment of the two outcomes cough and 'withdrawal' is provided (Box C8.4). This is because quality can vary between outcomes even if they are measured in the same studies. While cough is a subjective outcome susceptible to bias in the absence of blinding, the outcome withdrawal is objective and absence of blinding is unlikely to influence the count of people who withdraw. Lack of blinded outcome assessment would be a limitation of the study quality for cough but it would not be for counting the number of 'withdrawals'.

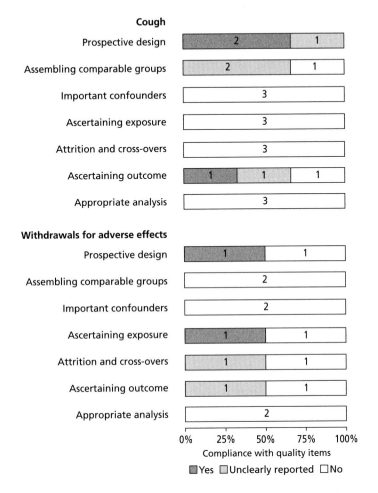

Box C8.4 Description of quality of comparative observational studies on adverse effects of angiotensin-receptor blockers (ARBs) *versus* angiotensin-converting-enzyme inhibitors (ACE-Is) in essential hypertension

Cough

Prospective design	2 / 1
Assembling comparable groups	2 / 1
Important confounders	3
Ascertaining exposure	3
Attrition and cross-overs	3
Ascertaining outcome	1 / 1 / 1
Appropriate analysis	3

Withdrawals for adverse effects

Prospective design	1 / 1
Assembling comparable groups	2
Important confounders	2
Ascertaining exposure	1 / 1
Attrition and cross-overs	1 / 1
Ascertaining outcome	1 / 1
Appropriate analysis	2

0%   25%   50%   75%   100%
Compliance with quality items
■Yes ▨Unclearly reported ☐No

This case study only describes the observational studies. Data in stacks represents the number of studies

Studies reporting on cough

The three cohort studies reporting on cough had considerable methodological weaknesses: Due to the observational design, all studies were open label; patients, healthcare providers and outcome assessors were aware of the treatment allocations except in one study where the telephone interviewer who did the outcome assessment was blinded. All studies lacked conclusive information about co-morbidities and co-medication. Most studies did not report on loss to follow-up.

Studies reporting on 'withdrawals due to adverse effects'

Two observational studies (one cohort study and one case-control study) reporting on 'withdrawals due to adverse effects', too, had profound weaknesses. While some quality issues, e.g. blinding, were difficult or impossible to address, others would have been amenable to methodological safeguards, such as the case-control study could have described its selection of cases and controls. Both studies lacked information about patient characteristics, co-morbidities, co-medication and adjustment for differences in prognostic factors. Furthermore, they reported that significant amounts of data were missing and there was considerable loss to follow-up.

Step 4: Summarizing the evidence
Cough

Three cohort studies reported on cough: one large post-marketing cohort study with more than 50 000 patients and two smaller studies with 449 patients and 49 patients, respectively. Among a total of 51 908 patients there were 691 cough events. The pooled summary estimate for ARBs to reduce cough compared to ACE-Is was an odds ratio or OR of 0.40 with 95% CI of 0.34–0.48. There was no heterogeneity in the effects across the studies ($I^2 = 0\%$; $ChI^2 = 0.80$; $p = 0.67$).

> **Odds ratio (OR)** is an effect measure for binary data. It is the ratio of odds in the experimental group to the odds in the control group.

'Withdrawal due to adverse effects'

One cohort and one case-control study reported on 'withdrawals due to adverse effects'. Both studies were small with 39 and 88 patients, respectively. The two studies with this outcome found 18 withdrawals in 127 patients. After pooling, the point estimate described a large effect and an OR of 0.36, but the 95% CI ranged from 0.12 to 1.08. Such a large spread in the confidence interval indicated imprecision arising from a small number of participants and a low number of events.

Careful readers might have noticed in Box C8.5 that results from the cohort and the case-control study designs are combined. Study designs have different weaknesses and potentials for bias and should not normally be mixed up in meta-analysis. There is agreement that the results from randomized trials and observational studies should not be pooled. How best to synthesize non-randomized studies of different designs (e.g. case-control and cohort studies) is an issue of ongoing debate. It is clear that pooling does not compensate for methodological weaknesses. One point of view is that if these weaknesses lead to differences in effects, which will be captured by an increase in heterogeneity. This should encourage the exploration of reasons for heterogeneity (Boxes 4.6 and 4.7).

What are the circumstances in which the results from observational studies are sufficiently compelling to warrant trust in their findings. Strong or very strong associations between exposure and outcome will be prerequisite. Some authorities recommend using an OR value smaller than 0.5 or larger than 2 to define a strong association or large effect. Although observational studies are susceptible to bias and confounding that lead often to overestimation of the effects, it is unlikely that imbalance of prognostic factors between comparison groups will be solely responsible for large or very large effects. Thus, intervention or exposure is likely to be contributing to the observed effect.

Step 5: Interpreting the findings

How can we bring together what we have learnt in the previous Steps to come up with a decision? Step 1 has ranked the outcomes of interest according to their importance for patients and introduced the distinction between patient-important and surrogate outcomes (the latter are regarded as indirect evidence for patient-important outcomes). In Step 2 studies have been selected taking study design into consideration. Step 3 has reviewed the methodological quality of the selected studies. Step 4 has explored heterogeneity of results and produced summary effects.

The gauging of strength of the evidence is shown separately for each outcome (Box C8.6). For the outcome cough the point estimate of OR showed an association. The 95% confidence interval around this estimate was very precise. In the absence of features that impair the strength of the overall evidence, such a large effect could increase our confidence that ARBs 'truly' lower the risk of cough compared to ACE-Is. Concerning 'withdrawals due to adverse effects', both studies reported fewer withdrawals for patients treated with ARBs compared to ACE-Is, but the estimation of association was imprecise. None of the five studies explored the effect of drug doses on the rate of adverse effect.

When assigning a level of strength to the evidence the starting point is the study design. The lack of randomized treatment allocation makes observational studies start at a low strength level. Methodological limitations of included studies relegate the strength to very low level. In this situation even large effects cannot justifiably raise the strength level.

The data available in the review on cough and 'withdrawals' from randomized trials was substantial. From 26 trials, the pooled relative risk, RR, for cough was 0.23 with 95% CI 0.16–0.33, indicating a strong effect resulting in less cough for patients treated with ARBs. From 21 trials, the pooled RR for 'withdrawals due to adverse effects' was 0.58 (95% CI 0.46–0.74), again indicating a strong effect with fewer withdrawals for patients treated with ARBs. Considering this information, the strength

The Grading of Recommendations Assessment, Development and Evaluation (**GRADE**) working group is an informal collaboration that aims to develop a comprehensive methodology for assessing the strength of the evidence collated in systematic reviews and for generating recommendations from evidence in guidelines. See www.gradeworkinggroup.org. Interpretation of findings in this case study draws on this methodology.

The **strength of the evidence** lies in the relevance of the outcomes, the methodological quality of the included studies, the heterogeneity of results, the precision and size of effects, etc, features that underpin the trust in the inferences generated from a review.

Relative Risk (RR) is an effect measure for binary data. It is the ratio of risk in the experimental group to the risk in the control group.

Box C8.5 Forest plot for outcomes cough and 'withdrawal due to adverse effects' comparing angiotensin-receptor blockers (ARBs) *versus* angiotensin-converting-enzyme inhibitors (ACE-Is)

Outcome: Cough

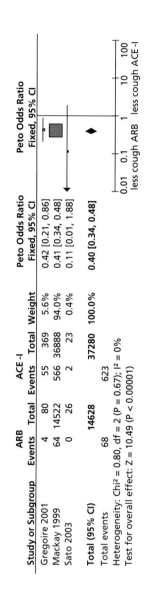

Study or Subgroup	ARB Events	Total	ACE-I Events	Total	Weight	Peto Odds Ratio Fixed, 95% CI
Gregoire 2001	4	80	55	369	5.6%	0.42 [0.21, 0.86]
Mackay 1999	64	14522	566	36888	94.0%	0.41 [0.34, 0.48]
Sato 2003	0	26	2	23	0.4%	0.11 [0.01, 1.88]
Total (95% CI)		14628		37280	100.0%	**0.40 [0.34, 0.48]**
Total events	68		623			

Heterogeneity: Chi² = 0.80, df = 2 (P = 0.67); I² = 0%
Test for overall effect: Z = 10.49 (P < 0.00001)

Outcome: 'Withdrawal due to adverse effects'

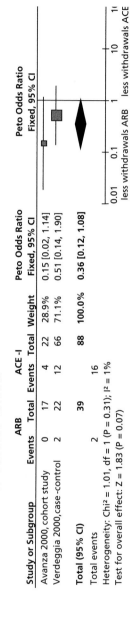

Study or Subgroup	ARB Events	Total	ACE-I Events	Total	Weight	Peto Odds Ratio Fixed, 95% CI
Avanza 2000, cohort study	0	17	4	22	28.9%	0.15 [0.02, 1.14]
Verdeggia 2000, case-control	2	22	12	66	71.1%	0.51 [0.14, 1.90]
Total (95% CI)		39		88	100.0%	**0.36 [0.12, 1.08]**
Total events	2		16			

Heterogeneity: Chi² = 1.01, df = 1 (P = 0.31); I² = 1%
Test for overall effect: Z = 1.83 (P = 0.07)

Review manager software used to compute effects and produce graphics.

Box C8.6 Assessment of the strength of overall evidence for the outcomes cough and 'withdrawal due to adverse effects' in observational studies comparing angiotensin-receptor blockers (ARBs) *versus* angiotensin-converting-enzyme inhibitors (ACE-Is)

Summary of findings

Importance of outcome	Outcome	Number of patients		Odds ratio (ARB/ACE-I) [95% CI]
		ARB	**ACE-I**	
Important	**Cough** 3 cohort studies Total events: 691	14 628	37 280	**0.40** [0.34–0.48]
Important	**Withdrawals** 2 observational studies Total events: 18	39	88	**0.36** [0.12–1.08]

Gauging the strength of evidence

Strength is initially assessed as low due to the observational study design. Methodological limitations relegate the level of strength of evidence to very low.

Outcome	Study design	Study quality (risk of bias)*	Size of effect+	Dose–response gradient	*Strength of evidence$*
Cough	2 prospective cohorts, 1 cross-sectional cohort	Serious limitations	Large and precise	Not available	*Very low*
	Initially assigned a low strength level	→ Relegation	→ No change	→ No change	⌐
Withdrawals due to adverse effects	1 prospective cohort 1 case-control	Serious limitations	Imprecise	Not available	*Very low*
	Initially assigned a low strength level	→ Relegation	→ No change	→ No change	⌐

* See Box C8.4
+ The methodological weaknesses of the studies were so serious that raising the strength level of evidence on grounds of large effect was not justifiable
$ Raised to moderate if not high level after consideration of randomized evidence. See Box C8.7
OR = odds ratio

level assigned based on observational studies can be raised to at least moderate if not high level. This increases the confidence that the rate of cough and of 'withdrawals' is 'truly' higher in patients treated with ACE-Is compared to ARBs.

Resolution of scenario

The overall summary of findings (Box C8.7) provides the basis for simultaneous considerations of both benefits and adverse effects of ARBs and ACE-Is in hypertension. This overview helps clinicians, policy makers and patients to balance their pros and cons in decision making. This review, including evidence from both observational and randomized studies, found moderately strong evidence that ACE-Is cause higher frequency of cough than do ARBs in patients with hypertension. In addition, more patients on ACE-Is withdrew from the clinical trials due to adverse effects than ARBs. From Case study 7 both drugs were shown to have similar effectiveness in controlling blood pressure. Armed with this information and the knowledge that ARBs are more expensive than ACE-Is, how would one decide? If the patient's healthcare insurance includes a co-payment, they would have to pay the cost of using ARBs out of their own pocket. Since cough is fully reversible after stopping the ACE-Is, the patient, in order to reduce cost, may decide to take the risk of adverse effects on ACE-Is first. Using the same evidence, another patient with different circumstances may make a different, but informed, decision.

Box C8.7 Summary of findings from a review on the comparative effectiveness of angiotensin-receptor blockers (ARBs) versus angiotensin-converting-enzyme inhibitors (ACE-Is)

| Importance | Outcome | Outcomes, study designs and results | | | Assessment of strength of evidence | | | | |
		Directness	No. of patients (studies)	Effect* (95% CI)	Study quality (risk of bias)	Inconsistency I^2	Imprecision	Publication Bias	Strength of evidence
					Beneficial outcomes				
Critical	**Mortality**	Direct	4264 (8 RCTs)	RR: 1.05 (0.40 to 2.75)	Some limitations	Consistent $I^2 = 0\%$	Imprecise	Not assessed	*Moderate*
	Stroke	Direct	1779 (3 RCTs)	RR: 0.84 (0.30–2.35)	Some limitations	Consistent $I^2 = 0\%$	Imprecise	Not assessed	*Moderate*
	Myocardial infarction	Direct	1628 (4 RCTs)	RR: 1.32 (0.54–3.57)	Some limitations	Consistent $I^2 = 0$	Imprecise	Not assessed	*Moderate*
	Heart failure	Direct	168 (1 RCT)	RR: 1.20 (0.68–1.78)	Some limitations	Not relevant	Imprecise	Not assessed	*Moderate*
	Renal function	Indirect Surrogates	499 (6 RCTs)	Effect Size 0.051 (−0.19–0.29)	Some limitations	Consistent	Imprecise	Not assessed	*Low*
	Successful monotherapy	Direct	4851 (19 RCTs)	RD (ARB-ACE-I) 0.00 (−0.02–0.02)	Some limitations	Consistent $I^2 = 0\%$	Precise	Not detected	*High*
					Adverse effects				
Important	**Cough**	Direct	51 908 (3 cohorts) 127	OR: 0.4 (0.34–0.48)	Serious limitations	Not assessed	Not assessed	Not assessed	*Very low*
	Withdrawals	Direct	(2 cohorts/case-control)	0.36 (0.12–1.08)	Serious limitations	Not assessed	Not assessed	Not assessed	*Very low*

● *Suggested reading*

This book focuses on core information about systematic reviews. The intricacies of many of the advanced techniques described briefly in this book, e.g. methods of meta-analysis, meta-regression analysis, funnel plot analysis, etc, can be examined in the materials referenced here.

Higgins JPT, Green S (eds). Cochrane Handbook for Systematic Reviews of Interventions. Version 5.0.0 (updated February 2008) The Cochrane Collaboration, 2008.

Available free at www.cochrane.org/resources/handbook/index.htm.

Egger M, Davey-Smith G, Altman DG (eds). *Systematic Reviews in Health Care. Meta-analysis in Context.* London: BMJ Publishing Group, 2001.

Fletcher RH, Fletcher SW, Wagner EH. *Clinical Epidemiology: The Essentials,* 3rd edn. Baltimore: Lippincott, Williams & Wilkins, 1996.

Glaziou P, Irwig L, Bain C, Colditz G. *Systematic Reviews in Health Care. A Practical Guide.* Cambridge: Cambridge University Press, 2001.

Systematic Reviews. CRD's guidance for undertaking reviews in health care. Centre for Reviews and Dissemination. York: University of York, 2008.

Available free at http://www.york.ac.uk/inst/crd/systematic_reviews_book.htm.

Mulrow CD, Cook D (eds). Systematic Reviews. *Synthesis of Best Evidence for Health Care Decisions.* USA: American College of Physicians, 1998.

Sutton AJ, Abrams KR, Jones DR *et al.* Systematic Reviews of Trials and other studies. *Health Technology Assessment* 1998; **2(19)**.

Available free atwww.ncchta.org/fullmono/mon219.pdf.

Guyatt GH, Rennie D, Meade MO, Cook DJ. *Users' Guides to the Medical Literature. A Manual for Evidence-Based Clinical Practice,* 2nd edn. New York: American Medical Association. The McGraw-Hill Companies, Inc; 2008.

Glossary

This glossary uses information from the publications listed in the Suggested Reading.

Absolute risk reduction (ARR)   *see* **Risk difference (RD)**.

Accuracy measure   A statistic for summarizing the accuracy with which a test predicts a diagnosis. There are three commonly used sets of accuracy measures for binary tests: sensitivity and specificity; positive and negative predictive values; and likelihood ratios. All these measures are paired. Single measures of accuracy are seldom used with the exception of the diagnostic odds ratio.

Adverse effect   It is an undesirable and unintended harmful or unpleasant reaction resulting from an intervention. It often predicts hazard from its future administration and warrants prevention or specific treatment or alteration or withdrawal of the intervention.

Attrition bias (exclusion bias)   Systematic differences between study groups caused by exclusion or dropout of subjects (e.g. because of side-effects of intervention) from the study. Intention-to-treat analysis in combination with appropriate sensitivity analyses including all subjects can protect against this bias. *Also see* **Intention-to-treat (ITT) analysis and Withdrawals**.

Baseline risk   The frequency of outcome in a population without intervention. It is related to the severity of underlying disease and prognostic features. Good prognosis is associated with low baseline risk while poor prognosis is associated with high baseline risk of undesirable outcomes. Baseline risk is important for determining who will benefit most from interventions. *Also see* **Number needed to treat (NNT)**.

Bias (systematic error)   A tendency for results to depart systematically, either lower or higher, from the 'true' results. Bias either exaggerates or underestimates the 'true' effect of an intervention or exposure. It may arise due to several reasons, e.g. errors in design and conduct of a study. This may lead to systematic differences in comparison groups (selection bias), differences in care or exposure to factors other than the intervention of interest (performance bias), differences in assessment of outcomes (measurement bias), withdrawals or exclusions of people entered into the study (attrition bias), etc. Studies with unbiased results are said to be internally valid.

Binary data   Measurement where the data have one of two alternatives, e.g. the patient is either alive or dead, the test result is either positive or negative, etc.

Bivariate model   A statistical method for generating summary estimates of test accuracy. It adjusts for the correlation that might exist between test sensitivity and specificity.

Blinding (masking)   Blinding keeps the study participants, caregivers, researchers and outcome assessors ignorant about the interventions to which the subjects have been allocated in a study. In single-blind studies only the subjects are ignorant about interventions, whilst in double-blind studies both the participants and caregivers or researchers are blind. Outcome assessors can often be blinded even when participants and caregivers can't be. Blinding protects against performance bias and detection bias, and it may contribute to adequate allocation concealment during randomization. *Also see* **Randomization**.

Boolean logic   Boolean logic (named after George Boole) refers to the logical relationship among search terms. Boolean operators AND, OR and NOT are used during literature searches to include or exclude certain citations from electronic databases. They are also used in Internet search engines.

Case-control study   A comparative observational study where participants/patients with the outcome (cases) and those without the outcome (controls) are compared for their prior intervention or exposure rates.

Clinical trial   A loosely defined term generally meaning to describe a study to evaluate efficacy and effectiveness of interventions. This term encompasses study designs ranging from randomized controlled trials to uncontrolled observations of a few cases.

Cochrane Collaboration   An international not-for-profit organization that aims to help with informed decision making about healthcare by preparing, maintaining and improving accessibility of systematic reviews of interventions (http://www.cochrane.org). The major product of the Collaboration is the Cochrane Database of Systematic Reviews which is part of the Cochrane Library (http://www.update-software.com/cochrane/). Those who prepare Cochrane Reviews are mostly healthcare professionals who volunteer to work in one of more than 40 Collaborative Review Groups (CRGs). Each CRG has a co-ordinator, and an editorial team to oversee the quality of their reviews. The activities of the Collaboration are directed by an elected Steering Group and are supported by staff in Cochrane Centres worldwide.

Cohort study   A comparative observational study where participants with an intervention or exposure (*not* allocated by the researcher) are followed up to examine the difference in outcomes compared to a control group, e.g. those receiving no care.

Comparative study   A study where the effect of an intervention or exposure is assessed using comparison groups. This can be a randomized controlled trial, a cohort study, a case-control study, etc.

Confidence interval (CI)   The range within which the 'true' value of a measurement (e.g. effect of an intervention) is expected to lie in a population with a given degree of certainty. Confidence intervals represent the distribution probability of random errors, but not of systematic errors (bias). Conventionally, 95% confidence intervals are used.

Confounding   A situation in studies where the effect of an intervention on an outcome is distorted due to the association of the outcome with another factor, the confounding variable, which can prevent or cause the outcome independent of the intervention. It occurs when groups being compared are different with respect to important factors other than the interventions or exposures under investigation. Adjustment for confounding requires stratified or multivariable analysis. *Also see* **Randomization**.

Continuous data   Measurement on a continuous scale such as height, weight, blood pressure, etc. For continuous data, effect is often expressed in terms of mean difference. *Also see* **Effect size (ES)**.

Control event rate (CER)   The proportion of subjects in the control group in whom an event or outcome is observed, in a defined time period.

Controlled clinical trial   A loosely defined term to describe a prospective comparative study for assessing effectiveness of interventions (regardless of whether randomization is used or not). Watch out for indiscriminate use of this ambiguous term in reviews. It is also a MeSH in the MEDLINE database.

Cost-effectiveness analysis   *see* **Economic evaluation and Efficiency**.

Diagnostic odds ratio   The ratio of the likelihood ratio for a positive test result to the likelihood ratio for a negative test result. It provides a single measure of accuracy. *Also see* **Accuracy measure**.

Diary keeping   A qualitative research method, usually an addition to questionnaire or interview data, where participants record experience and emotions contemporaneously. It can be free form, where people write what they want to, or structured where they have specific questions to answer or topics to write about.

Dose–response   A dose–response relationship demonstrates that at higher doses the strength of association between exposure and outcome is increased.

Economic evaluation (e.g. cost–effectiveness analysis) A study that takes into account both the clinical effectiveness and the costs of alternative interventions to address the question of how to achieve an optimal clinical outcome at least cost. The term cost-effectiveness analysis is often used synonymously but this is a misnomer. A full economic evaluation considers both clinical and cost outcomes whereas a partial evaluation may only consider costs without regard to clinical outcomes.

Effect (effect measure, treatment effect, estimate of effect, effect size) Effect is the observed association between interventions and outcomes or a statistic to summarize the strength of the observed association. The statistic could be a relative risk, odds ratio, risk difference, or number needed to treat for binary data; a mean difference, or standardized mean difference for continuous data; or a hazard ratio for survival data. The effect has a point estimate and a confidence interval. The term *individual effect* is often used to describe effects observed in individual studies included in a review. The term *summary effect* is used to describe the effect generated by pooling individual effects in a meta-analysis.

Effect modification It occurs when a factor influences the effect of the intervention under study, e.g. age may modify responsiveness to treatment.

Effect size (ES) This term is sometimes used for an effect measure for continuous data. *Also see* **Effect measure**.

Effectiveness The extent to which an intervention (therapy, prevention, diagnosis, screening, education, social care, etc) produces a beneficial outcome in the routine setting. Unlike efficacy, it seeks to address the question: Does an intervention work under ordinary day-to-day circumstances?

Efficacy The extent to which an intervention can produce a beneficial outcome under ideal circumstances.

Efficiency The extent to which the balance between input (costs) and outputs (outcomes) of interventions represents value for money. It addresses the question of whether clinical outcomes are maximized for the given input costs. *Also see* **Economic evaluation**.

Evidence-based medicine (EBM) The conscientious, explicit and judicious use of current best evidence in making decisions about the care of individual patients. It involves the process of systematically finding, appraising and using contemporaneous research findings as the basis for clinical decisions. Evidence-based practice (EBP) is a related term. Both EBM and EBP follow four steps: formulate a clear clinical question from a patient's problem; search the literature for relevant clinical articles; evaluate (critically appraise) the evidence for its validity and usefulness; implement useful findings in clinical practice, taking account of patients' preferences and caregivers' experience. Another related term is evidence-based healthcare, which is an extension of the principles of EBM to all professions associated with healthcare, including purchasing and management. Systematic reviews provide powerful evidence to support all forms of EBM.

Experimental event rate (EER) The proportion of participants in the experimental group in whom an event or outcome is observed, in a specified time period.

Experimental study A comparative study in which decisions concerning the allocation of participants or patients to different interventions are under the control of the researcher, e.g. randomized controlled trial.

Exposure A factor (including interventions) which is thought to be associated with the development or prevention of an outcome.

External validity (generalizability, applicability) The extent to which the effects observed in a study can be expected to apply in routine clinical practice, i.e. to people who did not participate in the study. *Also see* **Validity.**

Fixed effect model A statistical model for combining results of individual studies, which assumes that the effect is truly constant in all the populations studied. Thus, only within-study variation is taken to influence the uncertainty of the summary effect and it produces narrower confidence intervals than the random effects model. *Also see* **Random effects model.**

Focus group A qualitative research method. The collection of qualitative data using a group interview on a topic. Usually 6–12 participants are involved, and they can be used to gauge issues of importance. *Also see* **Interview.**

Forest plot A graphical display of individual effects observed in studies included in a systematic review along with the summary effect, if meta-analysis is used.

Funnel plot A scatter plot of effects observed in individual studies included in a systematic review against some measure of study information, e.g. study size, inverse of variance, etc. It is used in exploration for the risk of publication and related biases.

Generalization The extent to which findings of a qualitative research study are consistent with findings of similar studies, adding to the understanding of a phenomenon. Within qualitative research the aim is not to extrapolate to wider populations, so this term should not be confused with the terms External validity and Generalizability.

Generalizability   *See* **External validity**. *Also see* **Generalization**.

GRADE   The Grading of Recommendations Assessment, Development and Evaluation (GRADE) working group is an informal collaboration that aims to develop a comprehensive methodology for assessing the strength of the evidence collated in systematic reviews and for generating recommendations from evidence in guidelines. See www.gradeworkinggroup.org.

Guidelines   Statements that aim to assist practitioners and patients in making decisions about specific clinical situations. They often, but not always, use evidence from systematic reviews.

Hazard ratio   An effect measure for survival data, which compares the survival experience of two groups.

Health technology assessment (HTA)   Health technology includes any method used by those working in health services to promote health, to screen, diagnose, prevent and treat disease, and to improve rehabilitation and long-term care. HTA considers the effectiveness, appropriateness, costs and broader impact of interventions using both primary research and systematic reviews.

Heterogeneity/homogeneity   The degree to which the effects among individual studies being systematically reviewed are similar (homogeneity) or different (heterogeneity). This may be observed graphically by examining the variation in individual effects (both point estimates and confidence intervals) in a Forest plot. Quantitatively, statistical tests of heterogeneity/homogeneity may be used to determine if the observed variation in effects is greater than that expected due to the play of chance alone. For making a clinical judgement about heterogeneity, one might look at the differences between populations, interventions and outcomes of studies.

Homogeneity   *see* **Heterogeneity**.

I^2 statistic   It is a statistic for assessment of heterogeneity during study synthesis. Ranging from 0% to 100%, it gives the percentage of total variation across studies due to heterogeneity.

Intention-to-treat (ITT) analysis   An analysis where subjects are analysed according to their initial group allocation, independent of whether they dropped out or not, fully complied with the intervention or not, or crossed over and received alternative interventions. A true ITT analysis includes an outcome (whether observed or estimated) for all patients. *Also see* **Attrition bias and Sensitivity analysis**.

Internal validity   *see* **Validity**.

Intervention   A therapeutic or preventative regimen, e.g. a drug, an operative procedure, a dietary supplement, an educational leaflet, a test (followed by a treatment), etc undertaken with the aim of improving health outcomes. In a randomized trial, the effect of an intervention is the comparison of outcomes between two groups, one with the intervention and the other without (e.g. a placebo or another control intervention).

Interview   A qualitative research method. It involves questioning people about their views or experience of a phenomenon or event. Can range from structured, where each participant is asked the same questions, to unstructured, which consists of a list of broad areas to be covered, the exact format of each interview being determined as it progresses. *Also see* **Focus group**.

Inverse of variance   *see* **Variance**.

Kirkpatrick hierarchy   A classification of medical educational outcomes to capture the impact of educational interventions. It has various levels: 1a: Participation or completion captures attendance at and views on the learning experience, e.g. course evaluation; 1b: Modification of attitudes captures change in attitudes or perceptions, e.g. subjective reaction or satisfaction of participants with course, difference between pre- and post-course attitude questionnaire; 2: Modification of knowledge or skills captures change knowledge or skills, e.g. difference in scores from pre- to post-course; 3: Health professional's behaviour captures the transfer of learning to the workplace or integration of new knowledge and skills leading to modification of behaviour or performance, e.g. difference in performance after the teaching evidenced by more evidence-based prescribing and more frequent attendance at journal club; and 4: Change in delivery of care and health outcomes captures changes in the delivery of care attributable to the educational programme with or without assessments of improvement in the health outcomes and wellbeing of patients as a direct result of teaching, e.g. audit of practice showing greater compliance with evidence-based criteria.

Likelihood ratio (LR)   It is the ratio of the probability of a positive (or negative) test result in subjects with disease to the probability of the same test result in subjects without disease. The LR indicates by how much a given test result raises or lowers the probability of having the disease. With a positive test result, a LR+ > 1 increases the probability that disease will be present. The greater the LR+, the larger the increase in probability of the disease and the more clinically useful the test result. With a negative test result, a LR− < 1 decreases the probability that the disease is present: the smaller the LR−, the larger the decrease in the probability of disease and the more clinically useful the test result.

Mean difference The difference between the means (i.e. the average values) of two groups of measurements on a continuous scale. *Also see* **Effect and Standardized mean difference (SMD)**.

Measurement bias (detection bias, ascertainment bias) Systematic differences between groups in how outcomes are assessed in a study. Blinding of study subjects and outcome assessors protects against this bias.

MeSH Medical Subject Heading. Controlled term used in the MEDLINE database to index citations. Other electronic bibliographic databases frequently use MeSH-like terms.

Meta-analysis A statistical technique for combining (pooling) the results of a number of studies addressing the same question to produce a summary result.

Meta-regression A multivariable model with effect estimates of individual studies (usually weighted according to their size) as dependent variable and various study characteristics as independent variables. It searches for the influence of study characteristics on the size of effects observed in a systematic review. *Also see* **Multivariable analysis**.

Metasynthesis The amalgamation of the results of a group of qualitative studies on the same or a related issue. Included studies can be evaluated and the findings combined. This is achieved from reviewing the published data and not from meta-analysing data.

Multivariable analysis (multivariable model) An analysis that relates some independent or explanatory or predictor variables (X1, X2, ...) to an dependent or outcome variable (Y) through a mathematical model such as $Y = \beta 0 + \beta 1 X 1 + \beta 2 X 2 + ...$, where Y is the outcome variable Y; $\beta 0$ is the intercept term; and $\beta 1$, $\beta 2$, ... are the regression coefficients indicating the impact of the independent variables X1, X2, ... on the dependent variable Y. The coefficient is interpreted as the change in the outcome variable associated with a one-unit change in the independent variable and provides a measure of association or effect. Multivariable analysis is used to adjust for confounding, e.g. by including confounding factors along with the intervention (or exposure) as the independent variables in the model. This way the effect of intervention (or exposure) on outcome can be estimated while adjusting for the confounding effect of other factors. *Also see* **Confounding**.

Negative predictive value The proportion of subjects who test negative who truly do not have the disease.

Normal distribution A frequency distribution that is symmetrical around the mean and bell shaped (also called Gaussian distribution).

Null hypothesis   The hypothesis put forward when carrying out significance tests that states that there is no difference between groups in a study. For example, statistically we discover that an intervention is effective by rejecting the null hypothesis that outcomes do not differ between the experimental and the control group. *Also see **p*-value**.

Number needed to harm (NNH)   It is the number of patients who need to be treated for one additional patient to experience an episode of harm (adverse effect, complication, etc). It is computed in the same manner as NNT.

Number needed to treat (NNT)   An effect measure for binary data. It is the number of patients who need to be treated to prevent one undesirable outcome. In an individual study it is the inverse of risk difference (RD). In a systematic review it is computed using baseline risk and a measure of relative effect (relative risk, odds ratio). It is a clinically intuitive measure of the impact of a treatment.

Observational study   Research studies in which interventions, exposures and outcomes are merely observed with or without control groups. These could be cohort studies, case-control studies, cross-sectional studies, etc.

Odds   The ratio of the number of participants with an outcome to the number without the outcome in a group. Thus, if out of 100 subjects, 30 had the outcome (and 70 did not), the odds would be 30/70 or 0.42. *Also see **Risk***.

Odds ratio (OR)   An effect measure for binary data. It is the ratio of odds of an event or outcome in the experimental group to the odds of an outcome in the control group. An OR of 1 indicates no difference between comparison groups. For undesirable outcomes an OR that is < 1 indicates that the intervention is effective in reducing the odds of that outcome. *Also see **Relative risk***.

Outcome   The changes in health status that arise from interventions or exposure. The results of such changes are used to estimate the effect.

***p*-value (statistical significance)**   The probability, given a null hypothesis, that the observed effects or more extreme effects in a study could have occurred due to play of chance (random error). In an effectiveness study, it is the probability of finding an effect by chance as unusual as, or more unusual than, the one calculated, given that the null hypothesis is correct. Conventionally, a *p*-value of $< 5\%$ (i.e. $p < 0.05$) has been regarded as statistically significant. This threshold, however, should never be allowed to become a straight jacket. When statistical tests have low power, e.g. tests for heterogeneity, a less stringent threshold (e.g. $p < 0.1$ or < 0.2) may be used.

Conversely, when there is a risk of spurious significance, e.g. multiple testing in subgroup analysis, a more stringent threshold (e.g. $p < 0.01$) may be used. When interpreting the significance of effects, p-values should always be used in conjunction with confidence intervals (CI). *Also see* **Confidence interval (CI)**.

Performance bias   Systematic differences in the care provided to the study subjects other than the interventions being evaluated. Blinding of carers and subjects and standardization of the care plan can protect against this bias.

Phenomenon   An occurrence or a fact. Phenomenon is often used as a generic term for the object of a qualitative research study.

Point estimate of effect   The observed value of the effect of an intervention among the subjects in a study sample. *Also see* **Confidence interval (CI)**.

Positive predictive value   The proportion of subjects who test positive who truly have the disease.

Post-test probability of disease   An estimate of the probability of disease in light of the information obtained from testing. With accurate tests, the post-test estimates of probabilities change substantially from pre-test estimates. In this way a positive test result may help to rule in disease and a negative test result may help to rule out disease.

Power   The ability to demonstrate an association when one exists. The ability to reject the null hypothesis when it is indeed false. Power is related to sample size. The larger the sample size, the more the power, and the lower is the risk that a possible association could be missed.

Precision (specificity) of a search   The proportion of relevant studies identified by a search strategy expressed as a percentage of all studies (relevant and irrelevant) identified by that method. It describes the ability of a search to exclude irrelevant studies. *Also see* **Sensitivity of a search**.

Precision of effect   *see* **Random error**.

Pre-test probability of disease   An estimate of probability of disease before tests are carried out. It is usually estimated as the prevalence of disease in a given setting (e.g. community, primary care, secondary care, hospital, etc.) Sometimes, when such information is not available, it may have to be estimated.

Publication bias   Arises when the likelihood of publication of a study is related to the significance of its results. For example, a study is less likely to be published if it finds an intervention ineffective. Reviewers should make all efforts to identify such negative studies; otherwise their inferences about the value of intervention will be biased. Funnel plots may be used to explore for the risk of publication and related biases.

Qualitative research   Research concerned with the subjective world that offers insight into social, emotional and experiential phenomena in health and social care. Including findings from qualitative research may enhance the quality and salience of reviews.

Quality of a qualitative research study   The quality of a qualitative research study depends on the degree to which its design, conduct and analysis is trustworthy. Trustworthiness consists of several concepts including credibility, dependability, transferability, confirmability.

Quality of a study (methodological quality)   The degree to which a study minimizes biases. Features related to the design, the conduct and the statistical analysis of the study can be used to measure quality. This determines the validity of results.

Quasi-experimental (quasi-randomized) study   A term sometimes used to describe a study where allocation of subjects to different groups is controlled by the researcher, like in an experimental study, but the method falls short of genuine randomization (and allocation concealment), e.g. by using date of birth or even–odd days.

Random effects model   A statistical model for combining the results of studies that allows for variation in the effect among the populations studied. Thus, both within-study variation and between-study variation are included in the assessment of the uncertainty of results. *Also see* **Fixed effect model**.

Random error (imprecision or sampling error)   Error due to the play of chance that leads to wide confidence intervals around point estimates of effect. The width of the confidence interval reflects the magnitude of random error or imprecision. *Also see* ***p*-value**.

Randomization (with allocation concealment)   Randomization is the allocation of study subjects to two or more alternative groups using a chance procedure, such as computer-generated random numbers, to generate a sequence for allocation. It ensures that subjects have a prespecified (very often an equal) chance of being allocated one of two or more interventions. In this way the groups are likely to be balanced for known as well as unknown and unmeasured confounding variables. Concealment of the allocation sequence until the time of allocation to groups is essential for protection against selection bias. Foreknowledge of group allocation leaves the decision to recruit the subject open to manipulation by researchers and study subjects themselves. Allocation concealment is almost always possible even when blinding is not. Randomization alone without concealment does *not* protect against selection bias.

Randomized controlled trial (RCT)   A comparative study with random allocation (with allocation concealment) of subjects to interventions, and follow-up to examine differences in outcomes between the various groups.

Relative risk (RR) (risk ratio, rate ratio)   An effect measure for binary data. It is the ratio of risk in the experimental group to the risk in the control group. An RR of 1 indicates no difference between comparison groups. For undesirable outcomes an RR that is < 1 indicates that the intervention is effective in reducing the risk of that outcome. *Also see* **Odds ratio**.

Review   An article that summarizes the evidence contained in a number of different individual studies and draws conclusions about their findings. It may or may not be systematic. *Also see* **Systematic review** and **Meta-analysis**.

RevMan   The Cochrane Collaboration's software for review management and meta-analysis, available at http://www. cochrane.org/cochrane/revman.htm.

Risk (proportion or rate)   The proportion of subjects in a group who are observed to have an outcome. Thus, if out of 100 subjects, 30 had the outcome, the risk (rate of outcome) would be 30/100 or 0.30. *Also see* **Odds**.

Risk difference (RD) (absolute risk reduction, rate difference)   An effect measure for binary data. In a comparative study, it is the difference in event rates between two groups. The inverse of RD produces number needed to treat (NNT). *Also see* **Number needed to treat**.

Sample   Subjects selected for a study from a much larger group or population.

Selection bias (allocation bias)   Systematic differences in prognosis and/or therapeutic sensitivity at baseline between study groups. Randomization (with concealed allocation) of a large number of patients protects against this bias.

Sensitivity (recall) of a search   The proportion of relevant studies identified by a search strategy expressed as a percentage of all relevant studies on a given topic. It describes the comprehensiveness of a search method, i.e. its ability to identify all relevant studies on a given topic. Highly sensitive strategies tend to have low levels of specificity (precision) and *vice versa*. *Also see* **Precision of a search**.

Sensitivity (true positive rate) of a test   The proportion of those people who really have the disease who are correctly identified as such.

Sensitivity analysis Repetition of an analysis under different assumptions to examine the impact of these assumptions on the results. In systematic reviews, when there is poor reporting in individual studies, authors of primary studies should be asked to provide missing and unclear information. However, this is not always possible and reviewers often have to make assumptions about methods and data, and they may impute missing information. In this situation, sensitivity analysis should be carried out by involving a re-analysis of the review's findings, taking into account the uncertainty in the methods and the data. This helps to determine if the inferences of a systematic review change due to these uncertainties. In a primary study there may be withdrawals, so sensitivity analysis may involve repeating the analysis imputing the best or worst outcome for the missing observations or carrying forward the last outcome assessment. *Also see* **Intention-to-treat analysis** and **Withdrawals**.

Specificity (true negative rate) of a test The proportion of those subjects who really do not have disease who are correctly identified as such.

Standardized mean difference (SMD) Standardized difference in means is an effect measure for continuous data where studies have measured an outcome using different scales (e.g. pain may be measured in a variety of ways or assessment of depression on a variety of scales). In order to summarize such studies, it is necessary to standardize the results into a uniform scale. The mean difference is divided by an estimate of the within-group variance to produce a standardized value without any units. *Also see* **Effect** (erroneously called standardized mean difference).

Strength of evidence The strength of evidence describes the extent to which we can be confident that the estimate of an observed effect, i.e. the measure of association between interventions and outcomes obtained in the review, is correct for important questions.

Subgroup analysis Meta-analyses may be carried out in pre-specified subgroups of studies stratified according to differences in populations, interventions, outcomes and study designs. This allows reviewers to determine if the effects of an intervention vary between subgroups.

Summary receiver operating characteristics curve (SROC) A method of summarizing the performance of a dichotomous test, pooling 2 x 2 tables from multiple studies or multiple cut-off points. It takes into account the relation between sensitivity and specificity among the individual studies by plotting the true positive rate (sensitivity) against the false positive rate (1-specificity).

Surrogate outcomes   A substitute for direct measures of how patients feel, what their function is, or if they survive. They include physiological variables (e.g. blood pressure for stroke or HbA1c for diabetic complications) or measures of subclinical disease (e.g. degree of atherosclerosis on coronary angiography for future heart attack). To be valid, the surrogate must be statistically correlated with the clinically relevant outcome but also capture the net effect of the intervention on outcomes. Many surrogates lack good evidence of validity.

Systematic error   *see* **Bias**.

Systematic review (systematic overview)   Research that summarizes the evidence on a clearly formulated question using systematic and explicit methods to identify, select and appraise relevant primary studies, and to extract, collate and report their findings. By following this process it becomes a proper piece of research. It may or may not use statistical meta-analysis.

Theme   An idea that is developed by the categorization of qualitative research data under its heading. The large quantities of data produced by qualitative study are managed by the generation of themes and the coding of parts of the data to each theme. The perspectives of each research participant on each theme can then be compared and analysed.

Theory   Abstract knowledge or reasoning as a way of explaining social relations. Theory may influence research (deduction), or research may lead to the development of theory (induction).

Trial   *see* **Clinical trial**.

Triangulation   Triangulation is the application and combination of several research methodologies in the study of the same phenomenon.

Validity (internal validity)   The degree to which the results of a study are likely to approximate the 'truth' for the subjects recruited in a study, i.e. are the results free of bias? It refers to the integrity of the design and is a prerequisite for applicability (external validity) of a study's findings. *Also see* **External validity**.

Variance   A statistical measure of variation measured in terms of the deviations of individual observations from the mean value. The inverse of variance of the observed individual effects is often used to weight studies in statistical analyses used in systematic reviews, e.g. meta-analysis, meta-regression and funnel plot analysis.

Withdrawals   Participants or patients who do not fully comply with the intervention, cross over and receive an alternative intervention, choose to drop out, or are lost to follow-up. If an adverse effect is the reason for withdrawal, this information can be used as an outcome measure. *Also see* **Attrition bias**, **Intention-to-treat analysis** and **Sensitivity analysis**.

● Index

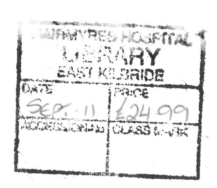
Systematic reviews

TO SUPPORT EVIDENCE-BASED MEDICINE

HOW TO REVIEW AND APPLY FINDINGS
OF HEALTHCARE RESEARCH

Khalid Khan, Regina Kunz,
Jos Kleijnen and Gerd Antes

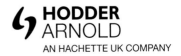 **HODDER**
ARNOLD
AN HACHETTE UK COMPANY

First published in Great Britain in 2003 by Royal Society of Medicine Press.
This second edition published in 2011 by
Hodder Arnold, an imprint of Hodder Education, a division of Hachette UK

338 Euston Road, London NW1 3BH

http://www.hodderarnold.com

Hachette UK's policy is to use papers that are natural, renewable and recyclable
products and made from wood grown in sustainable forests. The logging
and manufacturing processes are expected to conform to the environmental
regulations of the country of origin.

Whilst the advice and information in this book are believed to be true and accurate
at the date of going to press, neither the author[s] nor the publisher can accept
any legal responsibility or liability for any errors or omissions that may be made. In
particular (but without limiting the generality of the preceding disclaimer) every
effort has been made to check drug dosages; however it is still possible that errors
have been missed. Furthermore, dosage schedules are constantly being revised
and new side-effects recognized. For these reasons the reader is strongly urged to
consult the drug companies' printed instructions before administering any of the
drugs recommended in this book.

British Library Cataloguing in Publication Data
A catalogue record for this book is available from the British Library

Library of Congress Cataloging-in-Publication Data
A catalog record for this book is available from the Library of Congress

ISBN-13   978 1 853 157 943

1 2 3 4 5 6 7 8 9 10

Commissioning Editor: Caroline Makepeace
Editorial Manager: Francesca Naish
Production Manager: Joanna Walker
Cover Design: Helen Townson
Project Managed by Naughton Project Management

Cover image © amana images inc./Alamy

Typeset in 10 on 12pt Rotis Semi Sans by Phoenix Photosetting, Chatham, Kent
Printed and bound in the UK by CPI Antony Rowe

What do you think about this book? Or any other Hodder Arnold title?
Please visit our website: www.hodderarnold.com